Children's Pragmatic
Communication Difficulties

Children's Pragmatic Communication Difficulties

EEVA LEINONEN PhD
University of Hertfordshire

CAROLYN LETTS PhD, MACSLT
University of Newcastle

and

BENITA RAE SMITH MA, MACSLT
De Montfort University

W

WHURR PUBLISHERS
LONDON AND PHILADELPHIA

© 2000 Whurr Publishers
First published 2000 by
Whurr Publishers Ltd
19b Compton Terrace, London N1 2UN, England, and
325 Chestnut Street, Philadelphia PA 19106, USA

British Library Cataloguing in Publication Data
A catalogue record for this book is available from the
British Library.

ISBN 1 86156 157 1

Printed and bound in the UK by Athenaeum Press Ltd,
Gateshead, Tyne & Wear

Contents

Preface

For some time now people have recognized that children exhibit communication difficulties which can be described as pragmatic in nature. A great deal of ground-clearing has already begun and, in the past 15 years or so, we have learned about children whose difficulties seem to lie with the use of language in social interactions and/or connected discourse rather than with structural aspects of language (that is, phonology and syntax). There are children with known developmental disorders, such as autism, whose communication difficulties can be discussed in pragmatic terms, but there are also children who do not seem to fit neatly into diagnostic groups and whose difficulties can also be said to be pragmatic in nature.

The exploration of children's pragmatic difficulties is a challenging undertaking. There are some people who doubt that such difficulties exist separately from language or other developmental difficulties (Brook and Bowler, 1992; Gagnon, Mottron and Joanette, 1997; Boucher, 1998a; Bowler and Brook, 1998) and there are others who feel that there may be children whose primary difficulties are pragmatic in nature (Bishop, 1989; Conti-Ramsden, Crutchley and Botting, 1997). As Boucher (1998a) rightly points out, we do not know enough to be able to say for certain whether children exist with specific pragmatic impairments, given the lack of large-scale studies and problems associated with definitions of different developmental disorders. Our main aim in this book is to clarify what is meant by pragmatics, and hence, from the point of view of the field of pragmatics, we aim to explore what could rightfully be called pragmatic impairment. We are interested in how manifestations of pragmatic impairment can be found in data and how pragmatic theory attempts to explain them. We recognize that children (and adults) from many diagnostic groups manifest communicative dysfunction that can be described in pragmatic terms, and we will discuss the problems involved in identifying children with pragmatic difficulties in Chapter 8 (including a discussion on 'autistic spectrum disorders' and specific language impairment).

The field of pragmatics is difficult to pin down in precise terms, and equally contentious is the identification of indices of inadequate or problematic pragmatic development. This books aims to explore what it is that we know about pragmatic theory and normal pragmatic development and how this knowledge can be used in the exploration of children's pragmatic difficulties. We intend to explore how such difficulties can be examined and understood and how our understanding could be taken forward. Each chapter focuses on a particular aspect of pragmatic functioning which has been found to be problematic, or is potentially problematic, for children with pragmatic difficulties. For each topic, a theoretical grounding, supported by exercises and comments, is provided together with information about the development of that particular aspect of pragmatic functioning. The chapters involve relatively in-depth exploration of theoretical concepts, which are supported by more basic exercises and comments. We also explore what is known about language-impaired and pragmatically impaired children's functioning in the specific domains. Clinical data are used to illustrate pragmatic difficulties and interpretation of these data is given from both clinical and linguistic points of view. In this way each chapter conforms to a standard format: Key words; Background concepts and issues; Developmental notes; Clinical populations; Clinical data; Linguistic interpretation; Clinical interpretation; Summary.

Chapter 1:
Central issues

Key words: pragmatics, pragmatic impairment, appropriacy judgements, surface manifestations and underlying causes, cognition.

The aim of this chapter is to examine a number of central issues which underpin discussion in all subsequent chapters.

Key questions:
What is pragmatics?
What is pragmatic impairment?
What's in a name?
How to study pragmatic difficulties?
What problems are there with inappropriacy judgements?
What is the relationship between pragmatic and cognitive functioning?

Central concepts and issues

Examples of pragmatic difficulties

Before we begin to examine the above key questions, it may be useful to gain a feel for the types of difficulties that can be deemed to be pragmatic in nature. We will present two short samples of data here, which come from children who have pragmatic language difficulties and which demonstrate some of the difficulties we will be discussing in this book. We will provide only brief commentary on them here. The children's contributions that we consider problematic are asterisked.

EXAMPLE 1

This is Sarah (S) (aged 10;2) who is conversing with two adults (a research assistant 'A' and one of the authors 'B') while looking at photographs of A's horse. The discussion had veered towards zoos and is now coming back to A's horse.

B: Zebras look a bit like horses, don't they?

S: Yeah, but they've got stripes. They've got black and white stripes.

B: Umm. I mean [A's name] horse is sort of similar. Multicoloured.

A: Yeah. He has the same sort of colours.

B: But not stripy, but there is more than one colour you can see.

S: Oh yeah.

A: He has changed now. He's gone completely white.

S: Mmm.

B: Why do you think that is?

S: (laughs) Because I can see your horse is brown. (*)

B: Umm. That's [A's name] horse and that's another horse (points to the photo).

A: That's a friend's horse. Why do you think Jester's [name of A's horse] gone white? These pictures were taken quite a long time ago.

S: Oh, I don't know. He's really white there.(*)

A: He has got a bit older.

S: Yes.

A: You know how people's hair turns grey?

S: Yeah, that's when Daniel was a bit yellow but he's got much whiter now. About the same as that horse. (A and B did not know who Daniel was) (*)

A: Mmm.

B: Any other photos? No? I think the other children have gone out to play, you'd like to go as well, wouldn't you?

S: Yeah.

As this example shows, Sarah is very capable of conversing with the two adults. She provides both adequate and inadequate contributions. The main difficulty arises when one of the adults is trying, in a number of ways, to get Sarah to understand (or logically deduce) that the horse has gone white because it has got older and horses' coats, like people's hair, can turn white with age. To provide such an answer requires (minimally) the ability to conceive change over time, in terms of cause and effect (age causes hair/coat to turn white), and to appreciate that this is what the various adult contributions intend Sarah to work out.

EXAMPLE 2

These data come from Smith and Leinonen (1992: 262). Simon is 10 years old and is retelling a story without looking at the book (and pictures) which tells the story. Just previously he has told the story when looking at the pictures, producing more than 30 utterances, even though it was not possible for the listener to know what the story was about since narrative connections were left unclear.

> S: The people were walking on the snow. They walked on the mountain. All the people went up the mountain.

Simon then reread the story and looked at the pictures and then retold the story again without looking at the pictures.

> S: He went fishing. The boy went to bed. The people saw some sheep. The dog went up.

It is not possible to work out from these versions what the original story is about. It is about a boy who is asleep and is dreaming about the rescue of a sheep which is stuck on a mountain ledge. The first story has some internal coherence in that all the sentences relate to one another and tell us about some people who walked up a mountain in the snow. We do not know, however, who the people are or why they are going up the mountain. The second story is less successful, in that the sentences do not seem to be related to one another either in terms of time or participants. In this story, Simon attempts to cover a wider scope of the original story than in the first story, and this may have resulted in the less coherent structure.

Although recognizing that those interacting with the children in these examples may not provide maximally facilitative contributions, given the children's difficulties, it is our belief that each example demonstrates pragmatic (and related) difficulties that the children actually have. The initial realization is that the conversation with Sarah is not moving in the desired direction, or that Simon's various narratives are not coherent, and it is these kinds of realizations that lead to judgements of inappropriacy. We also believe that 'normally functioning' children of the same ages as the children in these examples would not have exhibited the difficulties apparent in these contexts. While reading these examples one needs to pay attention to the whole of the data, and to the intermittency of the children's difficulties. In Example 1, for instance, Sarah manages to answer some questions but not others. Such intermittency provides a valuable way forward for exploring the conditions in which the difficulties emerge and why. Similarly, exploring the question of why Simon's first story may be internally 'better' than the second story sheds light on Simon's difficulties.

What is pragmatics?

In broad terms, the study of pragmatics can be defined as the study of language in context. In the literature on both normal and disordered development, agreement is lacking as to what to include in the field of pragmatics. This confusion is partly a reflection of the state of the field of pragmatics itself. Pragmatics has focused on

(a) *Use of language in social interaction:* Here the focus is on interactional aspects of communication, including turn-taking, social and contextual constraints in language use and other conversational features.
(b) *Aspects of meaning not recoverable from the linguistic expression:* This includes implied and implicated meaning (for example, Grice's implicatures), intended meaning (speech and communicative acts), non-literal language (for example, idioms, metaphor and irony), referring expressions (for example, deixis, anaphora and ellipsis) and indeterminacy in meaning (for example, vagueness and ambiguity).
(c) *Connected discourse:* The focus here is on narratives and storytelling.

Sometimes, (a) and (c) are included in the field of discourse analysis, while (b) is almost invariably included in pragmatics. Without worrying unduly where the boundaries of the disciplines are, it is interesting to note that, at least on the surface, the areas highlighted here seem somewhat disparate. Their commonality, however, lies in the social and cognitive skills that an individual needs to use language appropriately. We will explore these skills throughout this book, which examines aspects of each area outlined above. There are dedicated chapters on conversational interaction, on speech and communicative acts, on narratives and storytelling, on referring expressions, and several chapters on implied and implicated meaning. In addition, many of the key themes cut across a number of chapters. We will cover both production and comprehension, but will focus primarily on verbal aspects of communication. This is not to say that non-verbal means of communication are not important, and particularly so in certain clinical populations, but simply to acknowledge our personal expertise in language and the constraints placed on a single volume. We will also demonstrate both data-driven and theory-driven approaches to studying the use of language in context.

One difficulty in defining pragmatics lies with the determination of where semantics (the study of meaning in language) ends and pragmatics (the study of meaning in context) begins. This has been a preoccupation of many pragmatists (see, for example, Levinson, 1983), and there is no definitive way of drawing the boundaries. For some, the delineation of semantics and pragmatics has become easier when working within the relevance theory framework of Sperber and Wilson (1995), which we will discuss in Chapter 7. In this account, fixed semantic meanings exist in quite a minimal form and hence construction of meaning in context (that is, pragmatics) covers areas of meaning one would more traditionally ascribe to semantics. These kinds of considerations gain significance in the context of children's pragmatic language difficulties if it turns out that what are traditionally considered semantic aspects of meaning may in fact be subject to pragmatic processing. Syntax is also touched by this issue of boundaries, in that aspects of language that can be described in traditional syntactic terms (for example, pronouns) are in fact pragmatic in nature in processing terms. In this way, more careful thought can usefully be given to what exactly we are testing, assessing and remediating when we focus on language impairments. We will return to these issues throughout the book.

Children's pragmatic impairments

Children can have both expressive and comprehension difficulties which can be described as being pragmatic in nature. The literature (for example, McTear, 1985a; Conti-Ramsden and Gunn, 1986; Culloden, Hyde-Wright and Shipman, 1986; Adams and Bishop, 1989; Bishop and Adams, 1989; Smedley, 1989; Bishop and Adams, 1991; Bishop and Adams, 1992; McTear and Conti-Ramsden, 1992; Bishop, Hartley and Weir, 1994; Vance and Wells, 1994; Shields et al., 1996a, b; Leinonen and Letts, 1997a, b; Kerbel and Grunwell, 1998a, b; Leinonen and Kerbel, 1999) has described pragmatically impaired children in the following terms. They

- have relatively good language skills (syntax and phonology);
- are willing to communicate;
- have difficulty with referential usage (making clear what, for instance, pronouns refer to);
- give too much or too little information;
- do not initiate enough or initiate too much;

- have difficulty modifying language according to the communicative partner (for example, formal and informal language);
- have difficulty noticing inadequacy in the information content of an utterance;
- have difficulty performing in open-ended communicative situations (versus more structured situations);
- have difficulty in using context to understand meaning;
- have difficulty in answering questions that require inferencing (constructing contexts) but do not have difficulty with descriptive questions (accessing context);
- have difficulty with abstract and imaginative concepts and have difficulty going beyond the here and now;
- are deficient in handling and integrating information for specific purposes. Have difficulty with drawing on world knowledge and with handling temporal sequences and cause–effect relationships;
- have difficulty telling coherent stories and producing coherent narratives;
- have difficulty producing relevant contributions in conversations (including relevant answers to questions);
- have difficulty developing and maintaining topics in conversation;
- are uncertain of the knowledge possessed by others;
- have difficulty with theory of mind tasks and right-hemisphere batteries and tests;
- have difficulty with idiom comprehension;
- overuse coping strategies (for example, no eye contact, minimal conversational contributions, frequent use of 'I don't know').

Not all children with pragmatic impairments would necessarily exhibit all of these communicative characteristics and not all of the time. Throughout the book we will focus on the kinds of difficulties children with pragmatic impairments have been identified as having, or can be predicted to have, and we will also comment on the children's communicative strengths. In the final chapter of the book we will discuss the status of pragmatic impairment as a diagnostic entity among developmental disorders, with particular reference to autistic spectrum disorders and specific language impairment. The current position is that there are children, without a diagnosis, whose difficulties are best described in pragmatic terms, but we are not in a position to say whether these difficulties are primary or secondary. We also recognize that clinicians in the United Kingdom are increasingly identifying children with 'semantic-pragmatic disorders', with or without autistic tendencies, and that more needs to be known about these children in order to provide appropriate intervention for them.

What's in a name?

We have already alluded to the fact that there has not been agreement in the literature as to how to refer to children's difficulties with the use of language. The labelling started with Rapin and Allen's (1983) 'semantic-pragmatic deficit syndrome' which was one of six subtypes of language disorder that they recognized (see also Rapin and Allen, 1987). This term suggests a clustering of difficulties rather than a more specific entity as would be suggested by terms such as 'disorder' or 'disability'. By this term Rapin and Allen refer to children, with or without an autistic disorder, whose language is relatively well formed but who have difficulty encoding and decoding meaning in a relevant manner in conversational situations. Rapin and Allen also use the term as a descriptive label that can be used across different diagnostic groups. McTear (1985a, b) talked about both pragmatic disorders and conversational disability and, in 1986, Stubbs asked whether there are disorders of conversation. These terms reflect the conversational difficulties that are likely to ensue from pragmatic difficulties. Bishop and Rosenbloom (1987) and Bishop and Adams (1989) have used the term 'semantic-pragmatic disorder', hence recognizing the close theoretical connection between semantics and pragmatics and the difficulty in disentangling the two. This term was initially most widely used by researchers and practitioners, even though it is presently losing ground. Bishop and Rosenbloom (1987) have also used the term 'high-level language disorder' to refer to children who have pragmatic difficulties, highlighting the fact that pragmatic functioning is likely to be connected with central cognitive processes (high level) rather than with a specialist linguistic processor (as in phonology and syntax). With the recognition that pragmatic difficulties may occur without semantic difficulties, the terms 'pragmatic disability' (for example, McTear and Conti-Ramsden, 1992), 'pragmatic impairment' (for example, Leinonen and Smith, 1994) and 'disturbance of pragmatic functioning' (Smith and Leinonen, 1992) were used. These kinds of terms are now most widely adopted and in this book we will refer to 'children with pragmatic difficulties' or to 'pragmatic impairment'. We will see these terms as describing difficulties which exist with pragmatic aspects of language without saying anything about underlying causes or clustering of difficulties. Bishop (1997, 1998) has now adopted the term 'pragmatic language impairment' (PLI), even though it is not entirely clear why. In some ways the insertion of the word 'language' can confuse matters further. The insertion of 'language' into the term cannot signal that pragmatic impairments are necessarily associated with language impairments, as data against this are presented by Bishop. Nor can it mean that when looking into pragmatic difficulties we are not interested in non-verbal aspects of communication, since these are intrinsically linked with pragmatic functioning and the identification of pragmatic difficulties (see Bishop, 1998, for Children's Communication Checklist).

Why have there been so many different terms for the same thing? This is partly a reflection of a developing field and the heterogeneity of the language-disordered populations in general, and partly of the difficulties involved with determining what the field of pragmatics covers. In some ways the history of pragmatic impairment can be seen in the names, and current terms may well yet change with our developing knowledge of children's pragmatic difficulties. There may well be subtypes which reflect different underlying causes or different surface manifestations. Leinonen and Letts (1997b) allude to this by referring to the possibility of 'inferential-pragmatic impairments', where a child's difficulty may lie with the inferential processes involved in comprehension.

Studying pragmatic impairments

Much research on children's pragmatic impairments has lacked explanatory power (for example, Bishop and Adams, 1989; Leinonen and Letts, 1997a). Descriptive research is valuable in the initial stages of research in a new field since we first need to know something about what the phenomenon is like before we can ask why it is the way it is. More recently, work has begun to look for explanations for surface difficulties, from within pragmatic theory (Leinonen and Kerbel, 1999) and from outside pragmatics (Bishop and Adams, 1992 – cognition; Shields et al., 1996a – social cognition; Leinonen and Letts, 1997b – inferential processing). Descriptive accounts without explanatory power pose difficulties for clinicians in the clinical management of communication difficulties. At other linguistic levels (that is, phonology and syntax), there is an argument that description of the difficulty a person experiences, together with a comparison with norms, is sufficient for the planning of effective intervention, but as abnormal pragmatic behaviour could be caused by a range of factors, which need to be addressed first, a comparative process is not likely to suffice.

Theoretical pragmatics and work on pragmatic impairments can be seen to differ in one main regard (leaving aside relevance theory, for the moment). The latter is concerned with real people, whereas the former is not necessarily so. Hence work with pragmatic impairments is intrinsically tied to processing factors, to views of mental representation and to theories of learning, as well as to consideration of other psychological factors (anxiety, confidence) and environmental influences (for example, the nature of input, opportunity to respond). Therefore, it is not possible to abstract away from reality, and consequently some theoretical pragmatics becomes difficult to apply. What is needed is a psycholinguistic approach to pragmatics and this is what we try to bear in mind throughout the book. We need to make a clear distinction between surface behaviours which can be described in pragmatic terms and different underlying causes that give rise to these behaviours. We need to bear in mind that different underlying causes can give rise to the same pragmatic difficulties and, potentially, one underlying difficulty can give rise to different surface manifestations. We subscribe to the view that pragmatics is both about description of surface behaviours and about explanation of how they came about. Such explanation can be viewed in two ways: first, explanation within a theory of pragmatics and, importantly, within a psycholinguistically real theory of pragmatics; and, second, explanation in psychological, cognitive, neurological or medical terms (or even genetic terms). Given our expertise and given what is currently known about pragmatic language difficulties in children, we shall concentrate on description and explanation in the field of pragmatics, but will, however, make connections with cognitive and linguistic factors, where possible, since explanation of pragmatic difficulties is intrinsically connected with these factors.

Some research on pragmatic impairment can be criticized for tending to focus on the child rather than the whole interaction. It has long been recognized that children's communicative functioning is affected by the nature of the input and the type of interaction s/he is taking part in (for example, role relationships, the purpose of the interaction). In the clinical context this raises issues such as what effect does the child's communicative behaviour have on other people and how should others modify, or not, their own communication with the disordered child. As we will discuss and demonstrate throughout the book, looking at children's contributions in the contexts in which they occur is not only very informative, but is a basic requirement for a pragmatic investigation. After all, pragmatics, by definition, refers to the use and understanding of language in context. The very defining feature of inappropriacy in language use is that the child's output is not adequate in relation to the demands of the communicative context.

The greatest challenge for research focusing on children, whose pragmatic difficulties seem to be primary, rests with the problems involved in identifying such children in the first instance. Research has relied largely on clinical opinion and thus circularity in research design is an unavoidable result. It is well documented (see, for example, Conti-Ramsden, Crutchley and Botting, 1997) that there is little agreement as to what characterizes children with specific language impairment and, for pragmatically impaired children, the picture is even murkier since there is not a clear view as to what could legitimately be called pragmatic difficulty and how such difficulties relate to various developmental disorders. Conti-Ramsden and colleagues' work shows that semantic/pragmatic disordered children were difficult to identify on psychometric measures and that it was clinical/teacher judgement of the children's difficulty which was the main factor in placing the children in the semantic/ pragmatic group. The conclusion is that we are yet to develop adequate psychometric measures for testing pragmatic functioning and in their absence many difficulties for research, assessment and diagnosis remain (see also Chapter 8).

(In)Appropriacy judgements

That a child has pragmatic difficulties has to be somehow identified. Identifying phonological, syntactic and, even, semantic difficulties is a reasonably straightforward task compared with pragmatics. This is because the first three have (more) determinate linguistic structures (and, even, rules) against which a comparison can be made. Developmental data are also more readily available for linguistic development other than pragmatic development. Pragmatic meanings are more fluid and indeterminate, being dependent on context. This is not, however, to say that anything goes and that there is no agreement as to what is inappropriate pragmatic behaviour and what is not. The point is simply that such agreement is potentially more difficult to find, given personal, social and cultural differences as to what is considered appropriate in given situations.

We see that we are in the business of making two types of inappropriacy judgements: those which are pragmatically more 'basic' and those which are based on personal, social and cultural views. Let us take an example of the latter type first. One of the authors was talking to a girl who was about 9 years old and was deemed to have learning difficulties. In the middle of this discussion, the girl stopped and looked at the author very intently (for what seemed like a long time). She then said: 'You should have washed your hair this morning.' The author defended her standards of hygiene by saying that she indeed had done so, but the girl insisted that the author's hair looked dirty. This kind of social inappropriacy is reminiscent of very young children who do not yet know the social and cultural norms concerning topics. This kind of inappropriacy can be seen to be different from that found in the two examples from Sarah and Simon that we discussed above. Sarah did not provide relevant answers to the two questions posed to her, and personal, social and cultural views are irrelevant to this decision. This judgement is made on the basis of the

specific contexts in which the questions were posed (see also Chapters 6
and 7). Similarly, the two attempts at a narrative by Simon do not count as
valid narratives because they do not have the basic features of a story (see
Chapter 5). This type of inappropriacy is more 'basic' to what pragmatics
is about than the personal/social/cultural kind. We are interested in
examining this 'basic' (in)appropriacy in this book.

There has been discussion of difficulties involved in making inappropriacy judgements in the context of children's communication difficulties
(for example, Letts, 1991; Leinonen and Smith, 1994). We believe,
however, that much more agreement can be found if we concentrate on
the basic kind of pragmatic inappropriacy rather than the kind associated
with personal, social and cultural norms. Leinonen and Kerbel (1999)
further demonstrate that working within a theory of pragmatics renders
inappropriacy judgements less subjective (see also Chapter 7). It is also
true that working in more specific contexts rather than in open-ended
conversational settings renders inappropriacy judgements more reliable
since the child's contributions can be assessed in relation to that particular context. Leinonen and Letts (1997b) found this very useful in their
investigation of comprehension of inferential meaning by a pragmatically
impaired child. To take an example from this study, we can see how the
specific context enables one to justify inappropriacy. In the following
example, Sarah (the same child as in Example 1, above) is answering an
adult question on the basis of a picture. In this picture two men are sitting
on a bench, having a break from planting trees. In front of them are two
trees freshly planted and a third tree that is lying on the ground next to a
hole, with spades and other digging instruments around it. The hole is
clearly intended for the tree which is on the ground.

> A: What is the hole for?
> S: I think it is for to put a treasure in it.

(from Leinonen and Letts, 1997b:44)

This is clearly an interesting and a creative answer in many ways, but it has
nothing at all to do with the specific context. As such, it is deemed
inappropriate. By identifying this inappropriacy (rather than trying to
make some argument for it being appropriate on the grounds of creativ-
ity), we can then ask such important questions as why Sarah would
produce this irrelevant answer, particularly when she has produced other
relevant and cooperative answers to other questions posed to her in this
task. It is important to be able to feel confident in making inappropriacy
judgements and this confidence is enhanced by specific contexts and by
working within a pragmatic theory. It is also important to make a judgement

about how a child construes the purpose of the interaction. If it turns out, for instance, that the child has decided not to play the game, but rather aims to entertain him/herself or others, then we cannot be sure if inappropriate performance reflects real difficulty. Our increasing knowledge of children's pragmatic development provides a further important yardstick against which to compare impaired pragmatic performance. More normative data are needed, however, for one to be able to say with confidence that a child's pragmatic performance is developmentally delayed or different.

Pragmatics and cognition

Throughout this book we will argue and illustrate that pragmatic functioning is intrinsically linked with cognitive functioning. Unlike linguistic processing (phonology and syntax), pragmatics involves integration of a variety of contextual and stored information for a specific purpose, and this integrative process is a cognitive process (for example, McTear and Conti-Ramsden, 1992; Smith and Leinonen, 1992). In other words, if one is processing for pragmatic meaning one cannot get away from cognitive processing. We will also explore the relationship between social cognitive functioning (such as the ability of one person to assess what the other person knows) and pragmatic functioning. In communication, we, as producers of communicative utterances, intend them to mean specific things, and those who attempt to figure out what we intend our utterances to mean will need to theorize about our minds (intentions). In this way, theory of mind abilities and pragmatic functioning are interlinked.

Future directions

In 1985, McTear identified the following as the key issues for future research (McTear 1985c: 124).

(1) Are pragmatic disorders related to disorders at other levels of language or are they quite separate?
(2) Are pragmatic disorders related to other non-linguistic disorders, for example, cognitive and social-interactional abilities?
(3) Is pragmatic disability a unitary phenomenon or are there several different types of disability which fall under the umbrella of 'pragmatic'?

Some 15 years on, these are still the key questions to be explored. Some progress has been made with regard to them, but a great deal of work remains to be carried out. These are important questions for the field to move forward from the uncertainty about the status and nature of children's pragmatic impairments. One aim of this book is to facilitate progress in our thinking and to help us clarify our positions with regard to such key questions as the ones outlined by McTear, and to raise further issues for exploration. Our ultimate aim, however, is to clarify and inform clinical thinking.

Chapter 2: Communicative use of language: speech and communicative acts

Key words: speech acts, indirect speech acts, felicity conditions, directives, communicative acts.

Aims

In this chapter we intend to look at individual utterances, not in terms of their syntactic structure or even in terms of the meanings of individual words, but in terms of the purpose behind utterances and the effects they achieve. This will be extended to consider how similar 'acts of communication' may work in the absence of language, and particularly in the early stage of development before linguistic communication is acquired. The following key questions will be explored:

Key questions:
How does language function as a way of getting things done?
What is the relationship between linguistic form and this effect?
What different effects can be achieved by using language in different ways?
Are there social and linguistic rules involved here, and what happens if they are broken?
What else is involved in communicating, besides language?
How does communication occur in the absence of language, or with only limited language?
How does the use of language develop?
How might this differ in children who are pragmatically impaired?

It will become clear how conventional ways of achieving results with language are only indirectly related to the form used. However, choices of words and forms will have an important influence on the success of this achievement, especially where the aim is to solicit help, cooperation or information from another person (and use of communication devices other than language may similarly affect outcome).

We will go on to consider the impact of impairment on the use of communication acts. An individual who is unable to manipulate forms or choose words in order to produce effective speech acts will be at an obvious disadvantage. Similarly, if the individual is unaware of the importance of making such choices then again s/he will be less likely to achieve a successful outcome.

Background concepts and issues

Why speech acts?

Consider the meanings of the following sentences:
(NB: Conventional punctuation has been omitted from many examples given in this chapter. This is because punctuation may influence one's perception of the function of an utterance. If a sentence ends in a question mark, there may be a temptation to interpret it as functioning to 'request information'. As we shall see, utterances with a question form do not always have a questioning function.)

(1) I promise to be there at nine o'clock
(2) I sentence you to ten years imprisonment
(3) I declare you to be man and wife
(4) I bet you £10 that it will snow today

In each case, the utterance of the sentence carries with it practical repercussions, in some cases profound ones, for the speaker, the listener or both. So in (1) and (4), the speaker is undertaking to carry out specific actions (in the case of (4) this is dependent on something else happening within the physical world). In (2) and (3) the repercussions apply to the listeners. These practical repercussions have nothing to do with language, other than the fact that language was originally used to set them in place. It can be seen that in instances like these, language is a very powerful tool. It was the philosopher Austin, in a book aptly entitled *How to do Things with Words* (Austin, 1962), who first noted that language used in this way was a purposeful act, performed with particular practical results in view. Austin used the term *speech act* to describe such an act. Of course, acts such as these work only under certain conditions. Utterance (2), for example, works only when it is spoken by a judge in a courtroom and, similarly, (3) must be uttered by a registrar or minister of religion in the right circumstances. Even (1) and (4) will not 'work' if the person uttering them is telling a lie or making a joke. Austin termed these kinds of conditions *felicity conditions*. Speech acts can be categorized according to type, for example, 'promising', 'marrying' and so forth. What then became apparent is that all utterances spoken in a communicative setting (that is, one that involves more than one participant and where language is used for communicative purposes) function as acts, although not necessarily with such serious consequences as the ones considered already.

EXERCISE 2.1

Look at the following sentences and describe the act that they perform. Then try to imagine the intention of the speaker, and any effects the act may have on the listener to whom the utterance is addressed.

(a) I declare this supermarket open
(b) Can you tell me what time it is
(c) Shut that door
(d) Well, I really enjoyed that

Comment 2.1

It very quickly becomes apparent that it is difficult to do this exercise in the absence of any information about context. For (a) we might imagine a scene in which a well-known personality is speaking at the opening ceremony of a supermarket, watched by a group of onlookers. The intention of the speaker is then to perform an act such that, from then on, the shop is open to the public, and the effect on the listeners is to realize that this is now the case. Change the situation to that of a bored manager opening up the supermarket in the morning and letting in the first shift of employees, and the effects are those of a joke or sarcastic remark. This emphasizes the fact that when any sort of speech act analysis is done, the context is of paramount importance. In the absence of context, as when looking at these artificial isolated utterances, the reader imagines some sort of canonical, or most common situation. Note that the meanings of the individual words do not influence this. We are not helped by the discipline of traditional semantics in making these pragmatic interpretations.

Assuming this 'most common' context, (b) is probably interpreted as a request for information and (c) as a request for some sort of action by the other person. This person must recognize these intentions in the speaker, that is to say that s/he is being requested to supply some information or to do something. Only when this has happened can the listener make up his or her mind whether to comply or not. Austin called the intention of the speaker the *illocutionary force* of the utterance, and the effect on the listener, the *perlocutionary effect* (with the utterance itself being the *locution*). In instances where there is a mismatch between force and effect, serious breakdowns in communication may occur. The speaker making a request for information (b), for example, may not seriously want to know the time (this would be a case of one of the felicity conditions for the 'request for information' speech act not being met), as in the case of the autistic child who is echoing an utterance heard earlier. Perhaps more commonly, the listener may not interpret (b) as a request for information, seeing it perhaps as an enquiry about his or her ability to tell the time. S/he may therefore just answer 'yes' without actually giving the time. Communication involves a successful match between both illocution and perlocution here. As will become clear, social conventions, such as the accepted polite way to request the time, have an important role to play.

A descriptive term for (d) is rather harder to find. The speaker is expressing a personal opinion, concerning his or her feelings about something that has happened, and there is also an element of using language for a social effect, perhaps expressing feelings of gratitude (again in the absence of context it is difficult to know). It is perhaps easiest to describe this as a comment, or giving information.

A final comment needs to be made about the grammatical structure of (b) and (c). You may have felt that, although both are requests of some sort, (b) is more polite than (c). (b) is posed as a question ('can you ...'), whereas (c) has the imperative form. A 'bald' imperative of this kind is often associated with 'giving orders'. This may not be a problem in a situation where the speaker normally gives orders to the listener (for example, military situations, or a teacher asking a pupil to do something) but has the potential to cause offence in other situations.

* * * * * *

Of course, when we look at conversations, even where we are involved and know the context, we cannot be sure of either the illocutionary force (or speaker intention) or the perlocutionary effect (or listener interpretation) of individual speech acts, since these are personal to the participants. People make assumptions about the nature of these based on experience of repeated social interactions. Where there is difficulty formulating these assumptions, as may be the case with pragmatic disorder, then problems of communication are likely to arise.

Speech act and linguistic form

Traditionally, the grammatical form of the sentence has been described in terms of whether it is declarative, interrogative or imperative. Declaratives are used to make statements, interrogatives to ask questions, and imperatives to issue commands. The structure of each of these types can be described in terms of consistent grammatical rules. In English, an imperative is formed with the infinitive form of the verb, and the subject is omitted. An interrogative involves verb-subject inversion and, more specifically, auxiliary verb and subject inversion, so that where there is no auxiliary verb the dummy auxiliary *do* is used. There may also be use of a wh-word. The following examples illustrate these forms with the verb *shut*.

Declarative:	I am shutting the door
Imperative:	Shut the door
Interrogatives:	Is he shutting the door?
	Does he always shut the door?
	Who is shutting the door?

It soon becomes apparent, however, that there is not a one-to-one correspondence between these forms and the *functions* (that is, speech acts) that they perform. A yes/no question, for example, can be asked using a declarative sentence form and a questioning intonation pattern, usually rising. This variation is particularly apparent when looking at the ways in which people formulate utterances that have the illocutionary force of getting someone to do something. Such utterances are called *directives* by speech act analysts, and range from a gentle request to a command. The following utterances are all directives:

Shut the door.
Would you mind shutting the door?
I want you to shut the door.

Only the first sentence has the imperative form associated with commands. Searle, who built on and developed Austin's theories (Searle, 1975), called speech acts that did not conform to the grammatical form associated with their function, *indirect* speech acts.

As suggested above, the choice of form in which to express a speech act is likely to be associated with rules of politeness (so imperatives may sound less polite than directives expressed by means of an interrogative structure). In fact, the form of a directive can vary in other ways in order to mark subtleties of this kind.

EXERCISE 2.2

Rank the following directives in terms of how polite they sound. Try to imagine a situation where use of each one might be expected.

(a) Pick up that package for me, will you?
(b) Pick up that package.
(c) My hands are full.
(d) Could you pick up that package for me please?
(e) Do you think you could possibly pick that up?
(f) Could you pick up that package for me?

Comment 2.2

Of the directives listed, (b) is a straightforward imperative and seems the most abrupt. In many situations this would be the least polite way of expressing the directive, and likely to occur where the speaker has higher status than the listener. High speaker status (for example, military commander, instructor, parent) in relation to the listener is one situation that sanctions a less polite form. In other situations, the listener may be perceived as rude or brusque, but there are some situations where this form would be acceptable. Examples would be between close friends who are in a hurry, or where the speaker temporarily takes on an instructing role (as in showing someone how to do something).

Expressing the directive using an interrogative structure, as in (d), (e) and (f), seems to 'soften' the directive, presumably because the implication is that a possible response can be 'no'. (a) consists of an imperative form plus a tag question, and this, too, has a softening effect. In fact, merely adding questioning intonation to the imperative in (b) achieves something similar. Further additions serve to soften the directive still further. These include the insertion of *please* and *possibly* and also the embedding of the directive as in (e) ('do you think you could ...'). However, the more 'softeners' are added, the easier it is to imagine that the speaker is being sarcastic. Speakers in this case would have the same status relationship to the listener as those using the straightforward imperative (b).

McTear (1985a) also points out that 'softening' of directives may occur between apparent equals (such as the two small girls playing together who were the subjects for McTear's study). In such cases this relates to what he calls the 'costs' and 'benefits' of the request (p.116). Where the cost of complying with a request is likely to be high for the listener (such as requiring the relinquishing of something that the listener wants to keep, or involving inconvenience), then the more grammatically complex, softer forms will be used. Benefits relate to the advantage to the requester if the directive is complied with. Where benefits are high, the requester is likely to use more indirect forms, and is less likely to accept a refusal without trying again.

Directive (c) is in the declarative form and at first sight may not seem to be functioning as a directive but as a comment. However, in the situation where the speaker needs to have something picked up, but has his hands full, he may well make this utterance with the intention that the listener does the picking up. There is a risk here that the listener may misinterpret the directive as a comment – that is, that the utterance would fail to have the desired perlocutionary effect. The listener may also choose to deliberately 'misinterpret' the speaker's intention if he does not wish to comply. Such directives are best described as *hints*. Reasons behind using hints (which, after all, carry a high risk of failure) are complex, and seem to revolve around issues of *face*. If the request is not complied with, there is no loss of face for the speaker (that is, he/she is not seen to be rejected), because there is no clear evidence that a request has been made. For further discussion of face and the use of hints, see Brown and Levinson (1987). Similarly, the listener is (in theory) not perceived as being rude or unhelpful by failing to comply, since he/she can argue that they did not realize that a request was being made. In practice, the situation would seem to be rather more complex, since judgements are made about failure to 'take' hints (as in: 'I told her I had a lot to carry, but she still didn't offer to help ...'). Speakers may use hints in situations where they feel they should not *have* to be explicit. Failure to comply may result in moral rather than linguistic judgements; clearly anyone who has difficulty interpreting indirect speech acts is in grave danger here.

*   *   *   *   *   *

It can be seen from this exercise that the choice of structure and vocabulary in making a directive is a delicate one. Important variables influencing the choice include status of hearer and speaker, and situation. It is difficult to specify the rules involved with any clarity. Whereas, for example, there is a tendency for abrupt imperative forms to be used where there is a difference in status between speaker and listener, these forms are also acceptable where speaker and listener have a close relationship and consequently there is less need to be polite. Any observable tendencies are effectively reversed when irony is involved. Cost to the addressee, regardless of status, is another variable that must be taken into consideration.

At the same time, the social effects of any mistakes are very real. People will spend time discussing why someone might have been unusually abrupt on any particular occasion, and also spend time agonizing over whether they may themselves have caused offence by saying something in the wrong way. For the child acquiring language, there are two main tasks. First, s/he must learn to express and understand speech acts accurately; that is, others must be able to interpret such acts correctly, and the child must recognize the speech acts of others. Second, speech acts, especially directives, must be expressed in a way that is socially acceptable in any given situation; the success of any directive will be largely dependent on this. We mentioned in Chapter 1 that social inappropriacy would not be the focus of this book. However, we can see that inappropriate selection of the forms of directives can have effects, first, on the listener's comprehension of the form as having the function of a directive, and, second, on whether this form disposes them to do what is asked. Potentially, difficulties in either of these areas will affect the outcome of any request.

Communicative acts

Speech acts by definition can apply only to spoken language. However, it is clear that similar 'acts' can be performed without using language, and also that non-verbal behaviour may supplement speech acts in important ways. Gesture and facial expression can perform functions similar to speech acts, and in the young child at the pre-linguistic stage these will be the only means of communicating. Such acts can be very effective.

EXERCISE 2.3

Describe the 'act' of communication an infant is performing by each of the following:

(a) Screwing up face while being fed. If pushed, spitting food out.
(b) Crying when hungry.
(c) Eye gaze in the direction of a colourful object, followed by pointing.
(d) Reaching for object and making 'whining' noise.
(e) Waving as familiar person walks away.

Comment 2.3

(a) and (b) are quite straightforward. In (a), the baby is expressing rejection, and in (b) attracting attention. It could also be argued that (b) functions as a directive to be fed. Both of these almost certainly initially are reflexive activities, outside the baby's control (and (b) probably remains so), but are relatively easily given an appropriate interpretation by a caring adult. Interestingly, these interpretations go beyond the provision of food and comfort, as we can see in (c) and (d). It is well documented that the adult will follow a child's gaze, and then very often comment on whatever has attracted the child's attention (see, for example, Harris, 1992). The child learns that directing gaze in this way functions to attract the adult's attention (*attention getting*), and to direct it towards the interesting item (*attention directing*); pointing is even more effective. The first frustrated attempt to reach for an object may again not have involved any attempt to communicate on the infant's part, but will have been interpreted as such by the adult. So the baby quickly learns that the behaviour in (d) will result in the adult fetching the object (if appropriate). Bates (1976) coined the terms *proto-declarative* for (c), and *proto-imperative* for (d). (c) is therefore seen as a preliminary to using language to comment on something (typically involving a declarative form), and (d) as a primitive directive.

(e), on the other hand, is almost certainly a behaviour that is initiated and 'taught' by adults. The child is unlikely to accidentally wave his hand and then discover that this is a useful means of communication. Waving goodbye is a social behaviour (in 'act' terms this would come under *greeting*), which the infant will learn to associate with departures through repetition of the action at these times and encouragement to carry out the action himself or herself.

* * * * * *

Pre-linguistic acts like those discussed above are important markers of communication development. They are also highly significant for those who work with people who remain at this stage as a result of learning disability or other conditions such as autism. Identifying and teaching behaviours that can function to indicate simple acts of communication for such people is very important.

At later stages in the normally developing individual, speech is likely to be the preferred medium of communication. However, gesture and facial expression still play a major role in modifying the illocutionary force of what is said (intonation, of course, is also very important). For example, a sentence such as 'how delightful' said with a negative facial expression (and probably flat intonation) is likely to be being used ironically, with the intended meaning of dislike rather than delight.

As any act of this kind clearly involves more than speech (and may not involve speech at all), the term *communicative act* (c-act) is preferred here to speech act. The c-act may not only be considered to include non-verbal communicative behaviour; it may also subsume notions of the impact of the act on the ongoing conversation or discourse (to be discussed in Chapter 3), as described by Edmondson (1981). Taken to extremes, the characterization of an individual c-act could also involve a complete description of the social and cultural environment in which the act takes place, plus the interactive history of the participants. (This approach is embodied in the work of *ethnographers* of communication. See, for example, Hymes, 1972 and Labov and Fanshel, 1977.)

Taxonomies of c-acts

It can be seen from the last paragraph that there is considerable variety in the way that c-acts are conceptualized, depending on the point of view of the researchers involved. Those writing about the development of c-acts in child language (for example, Dore, 1975; Halliday, 1975; Wells, 1985) have used a variety of taxonomies to describe the different communicative acts that children achieve. For example, Wells (1985), in his account of coding systems used in his seminal study of child language acquisition carried out in Bristol, describes five classes of 'conversational sequence' (p.62). These are classified according to 'the dominant purpose that they are designed to achieve', as follows:

> *Control*: the control of the present or future behaviour of one or
>   more of the participants.
> *Expressive*: the expression of spontaneous feelings.
> *Representational*: the requesting and giving of information.
> *Social*: the establishment and maintenance of social relationships.
> *Tutorial*: interaction where one of the participants has a deliberately
>   didactic purpose.
>
> (from Wells, 1985: 62)

These general classes refer to sequences of conversation which have a particular theme or purpose. Individual c-acts, or sequences of c-acts, can be used to make a *move* in a conversation, which may also be described in terms of having a particular purpose. (In the next chapter we will look in detail at how conversations are structured in terms of sequences of moves.) Wells describes how such purposes, or *functions*, develop (or, to use Wells' terminology, *emerge* in the sequence of development). For the *control* functions, a general category of *wanting* emerges first, and this is then elaborated into expressions of the functions *intend*, *request permission* and *prohibition*. Further functions develop on the basis of these three. The last groups of functions to emerge are *permit, threat, warning, promise, contractual* and *condition*, all of which, Wells claims, 'show the child beginning to use language to control behaviour at a distance' (Wells, 1985: 178–9).

This is just one example of an attempt to classify c-acts according to their functions (note that Wells draws on the earlier work of Halliday and Dore in formulating his own classification system.) It can be seen that such a system is quite complex, as functions develop from earlier broad undif-ferentiated categories, to functions that are much more sophisticated. Another feature that becomes clear when looking at taxonomies of this kind is that it is impossible to ignore the conversational and wider context in which c-acts occur. C-acts will take place in response to a situation, and will in turn be responded to by others.

Yet another issue that may become apparent at this point is that using a taxonomy to categorize c-acts is not easy. Clear criteria are needed for each category and the potential for disagreement is great. Where skilled language users are involved (think, for example, of language typically used by politicians), the listener may be unable to distinguish clearly between an utterance functioning as a threat, as a warning or as some sort of comment. While the perlocutionary effect might be such that the listener feels threatened, s/he may not be able to provide objective evidence that a threat was intended; the speaker can then achieve the possibly desired effect of threatening without anyone being able to accuse him/her of behaving in a threatening manner. When it comes to looking at unsophisticated speakers – that is, young children – plainly the analyst is aided by context and knowledge of the child. It is important, then, to include as much detail as possible concerning context and background information when carrying out any analysis of c-act use. The following exercise illustrates some of these issues.

EXERCISE 2.4

Three-year-old Carl(C) has a mild general developmental delay and a more severe delay in communication skills. His language output is limited to single words. His speech and language therapist (T) is setting up an activity where he searches for items hidden around the room. First, though, he is asked to 'hide his eyes', while she hides the items. His mother (M) is helping with this.

M: (tries to get C to close his eyes, by placing her hand over them)
C: (pushes M's hands away)
C: (points to items he can see T placing around the room)
there, there, there

(NB: Actions and contextual features are given in brackets)

Can you describe the c-acts that C is performing by both his actions and his words?

Comment on 2.4

The first consideration is what communicative value to put on C's non-verbal actions. The action of pushing his mother's hands away can be interpreted as merely reflexive, a response to discomfort, or as communicating a refusal to close his eyes or cooperate in the activity. If the last interpretation is adopted, then this action constitutes a c-act expressing something like 'refusal'.

In the second part of C's contribution to this interaction, he accompanies repetition of the word 'there' with a pointing gesture. At one level this could be interpreted as serving the function of drawing attention to the items being placed around the room, some sort of 'attention getter' or 'comment'. However if it is felt that C knows that he is supposed not to see where the items are being placed, then rather more can be read into this c-act, in terms of expressing defiance and a general desire not to cooperate.

Some additional background knowledge helps here. C at this stage had a very limited attention span, and quickly tired of any activity. Immediately preceding this extract he had seemed to comply with the suggestion that he 'hide his eyes', by sitting still with his eyes closed. A reasonable interpretation of his action of pushing away his mother's hands would be that of a refusal, C having had enough of trying to keep his eyes closed. His second c-act is not so straightforward. C at this stage frequently failed to cooperate with tasks, preferring to follow his own agenda. He had also played the 'finding' game before, so possibly knew the purpose behind closing his eyes. Whether this lack of willingness to go along with the activity can be interpreted as 'defiance', though, is open to question and clearly cannot be ascertained without knowing exactly what C was thinking and feeling at the time. This brings into focus issues concerning the motivation behind uncooperative behaviour. Is C's attention span too limited to cope with this activity, or is he deliberately setting out to be difficult? If the latter, is it the case that he does not enjoy the activity, finds it boring (perhaps because he has done it before) or has something happened prior to the session to upset him?

You may have found that you placed different interpretations on C's behaviour here. You may have revised your interpretations in the light of the additional background knowledge given later, but you may not have done, or you may have come to a new set of different interpretations. For example, you may have decided that Carl's behaviour in pushing away his mother's hand and drawing attention to things around the room is the result of eagerness to get on with an activity he enjoys; he does not realize how long it takes to set up the items for the activity, or he thinks the therapist is being unreasonably slow. In this case, the therapist might conclude that the activity is a motivating one, but that she needs to take steps to set it up before Carl arrives.

* * * * * *

This range of plausible interpretations highlights one of the major problems encountered when trying to do any sort of pragmatic analysis. Because inferences have to be made about people's feelings and intentions (and frequently this may be after the event, when analysing recorded or transcribed data), researchers may well not agree on the categorization of any particular c-act or sequence. Difficulties of *inter-rater reliability* therefore tend to arise when any analysis of this kind is carried out.

Developmental notes on c-acts

It can be seen from Exercise 2.3 that the genesis of c-acts is very early, and that they grow out of early reflexive actions such as crying when hungry. Coupe and Goldbart (1988) give an account of early pre-speech c-acts, from the earliest time when caregivers attribute meaning to a range of actions and vocalizations on the part of the infant, through use of proto-communicative acts, to the first words stage. The tendency for caring adults to read communicative meaning into the infant's cries and gestures is important in helping him or her to learn about the perlocutionary effects of communication that, in the first instance, may have no intended illocution. McLaughlin (1998) gives a vivid account of this in his book on language acquisition.

The next stage is to bring spoken language into the process, so that, increasingly, c-acts are carried out using language accompanied by appropriate non-verbal gestures and facial expression. From this point, not only is the range of c-acts available to the child extended, but s/he expresses them through a wider variety of increasingly sophisticated forms. McTear and Conti-Ramsden (1992) sum up the sorts of knowledge applied to the use of speech acts as follows:

> linguistic knowledge of how particular structures can be used to perform certain functions;
> social knowledge of the contextual considerations that determine the appropriate situations for the use of a speech act;
> sociocognitive knowledge that guides the choice of a particular form of a speech act on the basis of perceived characteristics of the listener.

(McTear and Conti-Ramsden 1992: 91)

In order to develop this sort of knowledge, the child must of course receive appropriate input from those in the day-to-day environment, who must ensure that models are supplied of how communication works and give suitable feedback to reinforce and consolidate developmental gains.

A useful way to become familiar with normal patterns of pragmatic development is to look at an assessment profile devised by Dewart and Summers (1995). Their *Pragmatics Profile* is an assessment procedure for documenting pragmatic skills and is used widely by speech and language therapists. It is carried out by means of an interview with parents or other carers; in this way the problem of accurate analysis of pragmatic behaviours posed above is to some extent mitigated by the fact that those making the analysis know the child very well. Parents or carers are asked questions about the child's communication in specific situations. If they are unable to think what the child does, prompts are used to help them make a judgement.

Summaries at the beginning of the profile give an overview of pragmatic development, including the development of c-acts, here considered under the heading of Communicative Functions. This section outlines first, at what point the child is capable of realizing certain types of act (and uses them routinely), and second, how these acts are realized in terms of gesture, language or both, again at different stages of development. So, for example, the 9–18 month period (in normally developing children) is characterized by ability to seek attention; request objects, action or information; reject or protest; express greetings; name items. This is done 'first by gesture combined with vocalization and then by words' (Dewart and Summers, 1995:6). Single or multi-word utterances begin to be used for some functions between 18 months and 3 years of age, while at 3–4 years the child can begin to use modal forms (for example, 'would you', 'can you' plus the request itself) to soften requests. Between 4 and 7 years, the child 'learns to express intentions in a variety of forms to fit the communicative needs of the listener and politeness constraints'. Functions expressed now include, among others, 'state rules', 'negotiate and bargain', 'taunt and threaten' (Dewart and Summers, 1995: 6).

As explained above, parents or carers are asked specific questions about how the child communicates various functions. If the parent is uncertain, examples are given as prompts. For example, when exploring the child's ability to 'Request assistance', the question is asked: 'If [*child's name*] needs help with something [*he/she*] is doing, how does [*he/she*] usually let you know?'

If the respondent is uncertain, suggested examples are:

Beckons or points to what is required.
Requests help but does not explain the problem.
Requests help and explains what is needed.
Gets angry and distressed without asking for help.
Waits passively.

(from Dewart and Summers, 1995, p.2 of Pragmatics Profile pro-forma)

In using a guided interview approach, the profile draws on the parent or carer's intimate knowledge of the child, and their experience of the child's attempts to communicate over repeated occasions. It can be inferred here that the third suggestion ('requests help and explains what is needed') is the most mature, whereas the first two are less developed. The last two possibilities could be interpreted (especially in the context of a number of maladaptive pragmatic behaviours), as being more abnormal and perhaps the behaviour of an autistic or pragmatically impaired child. Although the profile is designed as an assessment procedure, the summaries at the beginning and the different suggestions given to help interviewees answer the different questions provide helpful yardsticks for development.

Further useful insights into pragmatic development are provided by McTear (1985a). He describes the development of request sequences in two young girls who regularly played together, over a period of time between about 4;00 and 6;00 years of age. He notes that the children did not show a development over time from using direct to using indirect requests (instead they were able to use both on all occasions that recordings were made), but suggests that this is a feature of the peer-play situation, where direct imperative forms are frequently appropriate. He does, however, note the use (in all recorded sessions) of embedded imperatives, typically involving modals ('will you', 'would you' plus the request) and resulting in an interrogative form. These appear to be related to the 'costs' (see above) of compliance to the requestee; requests involving high costs were more likely to be mitigated by the use of an embedded form.

It is also noted that the children showed awareness of *meaning factors* (the term is taken from Garvey, 1975). These are the 'conditions underlying speech acts' (McTear, 1985a: 108), and correspond to felicity conditions mentioned earlier. The children would reinforce their requests by giving reasons for making them, such as their desire or need for something. Similarly, they could also refer to meaning factors as reasons to refuse to comply with a request. In the first recorded session the need for requests was questioned, and also the listener's obligation to comply. Other factors were addressed for the first time in subsequent sessions; for example, in the last session (children aged 5;01 and 5;05) reference was made for the first time to consequences of compliance and to the listener's willingness to comply. It is suggested that the children's awareness of conditions developed over time.

In order to gain an overview of the development and increasing sophistication of c-acts, the reader is referred to the chapter on pragmatic development in Andersen-Wood and Smith (1997), with particular reference to function/intentional communication, and also to the section on speech acts in the developmental chapter in McTear and Conti-Ramsden (1992).

Language impairment and communicative acts

When considering how impaired language may be reflected in the use of communicative acts, two main approaches are taken. To some extent, these reflect issues of language delay, where the child's communication is similar to that of a younger child, versus issues of language disorder, where the child's use of c-acts is qualitatively different from both the younger child and from age peers. In the first (delayed) case, it is possible to detect either a decreased range of c-acts at the child's disposal, so that some of the later-developing acts are not expressed, or a delay in the means of expression, or both. If means of expression are delayed, c-acts would be expressed by gesture or very limited language where more sophisticated forms would normally be expected. Underlying factors relating to such delays have to be considered carefully. It has already been pointed out that the child is dependent on linguistic development (at the levels of vocabulary and syntax), and on cognitive development in order to be able to deploy a range of c-acts successfully and that s/he also needs an appropriate level of social knowledge. It also has to be remembered that it may not be possible to interpret the child's intended c-act, if his/her means of expressing it are very limited. Finally, it must be borne in mind that the child may possess the requisite skills and abilities to perform a range of c-acts, but may lack the confidence or opportunity to do so in certain situations; the greater the number of these situations that the child experiences, the harder will be the impact. Some of these factors are exemplified in the further clinical examples to be given in this chapter.

To take the more disordered case, it is also possible that a child may express a c-act in such an unusual way that the addressee fails to recognize which c-act is being communicated. For example, the child may attempt to attract an adult's attention by standing close to them, or by staring intently. In a context where there are other children around and quite a lot is happening (a typical nursery school, for example), these attempts may go unnoticed, whereas calling someone's name or pulling on their clothing might be more effective. Willcox and Mogford-Bevan (1995) give an interesting account of two children (attending a school for language impaired children) who attempt to give directives by using a declarative form. Other children do not interpret these utterances as directives and so they are rarely responded to. Willcox and Mogford-Bevan's conclusions are based on extensive observation of the children interacting in a number of different settings and with different participants, and data were recorded using both video and pen-and-paper notes. Where a child's communication behaviour is bizarre, it may require extensive observations in different environments in order to identify patterns of this kind.

Felicity conditions have already been mentioned as conditions under which speech acts will have the desired function. Disordered children may use c-acts without the felicity conditions for their use being met. Bishop and Adams (1989) describe *inappropriate questioning* as one type of pragmatic problem (p.255). Such a question might be one where the adult could not possibly know the answer (breaking the condition that the questioner must believe that the listener will be able to supply an answer), or one where the child already knows the answer (breaking the condition that the questioner should need to have an answer, that is to say, does not know the answer already). It is often noted that very young children use questioning in this way, perhaps as a means of prolonging a rewarding interaction with an adult. The disordered child, however, will display this behaviour at a later age, and here it seems to be motivated by a strong need to control the conversation (see Chapter 3).

Fey and Leonard (1983) summarize some of the literature that explores the question of whether a specific language impairment (SLI) results in impairment of performance of speech acts. They note that this area is of special interest 'because of the partial interdependence between a speech act and the linguistic forms with which it can be expressed' (p.71). Studies reported are contradictory concerning SLI children's ability to use a range of speech acts, and some of the confusion may arise from the difficulties of keeping functional acts separate from constraints imposed by limited syntax or vocabulary.

The paper also considers SLI children's comprehension of speech acts expressed by others and there is some suggestion that this may also be impaired. This is certainly another aspect that needs to be considered. Evidence for successful comprehension of c-acts can generally only be ascertained from a child's response to any act that seems to specifically require one (for example, a directive). However, failure to respond correctly or 'appropriately' may be the result of any of several possibilities, including the following:

(1) The child does not understand the lexical items used.
(2) The child is confused by the length and/or complexity of the utterance.
(3) The child cannot deduce the illocutionary force of the utterance, especially where indirect speech acts are used. (An early study by Ervin-Tripp (1976) shows how young children, on answering the phone, are not able to work out what is required by a question such as 'Is your mother there?' They may respond with 'yes', but make no attempt to fetch their mother or attract her attention.)
(4) The child may not wish to respond in the desired way.

Assessment of c-act use by the child can be carried out using the Dewart and Summers (1995) profile already mentioned. An assessment by Shulman (1985), which is described by King (1989) and McTear and Conti-Ramsden (1992), also focuses on illocutionary acts. In this case a more structured situation is set up using puppets, and the child is stimulated through role-play to produce various act-types. This assessment has the advantage that it is standardized (using a sample of 650 children aged from 3;00 to 8;11). A disadvantage is that it may be difficult to elicit naturalistic c-acts from a child in a structured testing situation (criticisms of this test are summarized by Smith and Leinonen, 1992).

Clinical data

These data have been divided into a number of short sections which will be interpreted in turn. They are all from the same session with Carl, described in Exercise 2.4.

EXERCISE 2.5

Consider again what Carl may be intending to communicate through his actions and utterances. How are these c-acts expressed?

T is sorting through a pile of pictures, and showing them to C. C's attention is caught by a picture of a pair of spectacles. Both C's mother and T are wearing spectacles.

        T: do you know what they are?
        C: (points at picture, whispers) X
        T: who wears them?
        C: (picks up picture, points to it) ?Mummy
             (points to T)
        T: I do and who else?
        C: (points to picture) ?on there
             (points to mother)
        T: they're just like Mummy's aren't they
        C: mine (holds card tightly, away from T)
        T: no, I'll keep that one
        C: (throws card on floor)

(X = unintelligible syllable, ? before an utterance indicates that transcription is uncertain)

Comment on Exercise 2.5: Linguistic

C says very little in this interaction, and on two occasions it is not clear exactly what he has said. However, by means of non-verbal behaviour he indicates his interest in the picture and, with the help of some prompting, the reasons for this interest: he can match the picture with items worn by two other people in the room, especially his mother. He indicates very firmly his wish to keep the card, both with the word *mine* and gesture, but his annoyance at having it taken away is expressed entirely non-verbally – by throwing it on the floor.

Comment on Exercise 2.5: Clinical implications

It can be seen that a potentially rewarding interaction begins here, when C's own expressed interest is followed up. C is able to express this interest, albeit with only very limited verbal resources. Similar 'matching' situations (for example, where pictures show items of clothing that people in the room may have) may provide useful opportunities for developing C's interaction with others.

C is able to verbally express a desire to retain the picture, and reacts negatively when it is taken from him. It may be helpful to him at this stage to reinforce his communicative attempts here by allowing him to hang on to the picture (there can be little doubt that at this point C's common experience was to have many of his directive utterances thwarted, since they frequently did not match with what the adults around him felt to be appropriate). He is unable to think ahead and consider that the picture might be used instead in a (potentially) rewarding activity. This 'here and now' orientation, and extreme reaction when thwarted, is typical of a younger child (compare with a 2-year-old having a tantrum). Eventually, however, it will be necessary for C to move on from this orientation if he is to be able to participate in longer interactional sequences. The therapist will need to decide at what point she can make stronger demands on C, but this process will undoubtedly be helped by gaining C's confidence and interest through reinforcement, where practical, of his current communicative attempts.

Exercise 2.6

This time, think about the c-acts that the therapist is producing. Does Carl show evidence of understanding them?

Carl and T are playing a game involving threading coloured balls on to a stick. Carl has to wait until T says 'go' before placing the ball. He has been doing this fairly successfully. T tries to change roles, by getting C to tell her when to 'go'. C's father, D, is also present.

> T: (holding ball) can I have a go?
> You tell me
> C: (looks at T)

T: when shall I put it
C: (continues to look at T)
T: tell me
      ready...
      *go
C: *mine (tries to take ball from T)

T: are you going to tell me this time?
D: you say go, C
C: (takes ball, does not look at T or D) mine

(*indicates that both syllables were said at the same time)

Comment on Exercise 2.6: Linguistic

C gives no indication of understanding the instructions given by both T and D. He responds by using the word 'mine' to indicate that he wants the ball.

Comment on Exercise 2.6: Clinical implications

Although it may be the case that C simply fails to understand the linguistic contents of the suggestions that he give the instruction to wait (expressed on the whole very simply: for example, 'you tell me', 'you say go'), it is also possible that he is unable to switch roles in this way and use directives to command others, except to the limited extent that 'mine' is used to express the wish to keep hold of something. If this is the case, his ability to use communication to control others is obviously very limited, probably restricted to expressing pleasure or displeasure in response to what others do (although he has shown that he is capable of attracting another person's attention to something). The power of directive language needs to be shown to him, by creating situations where he can issue directives that will influence someone else's behaviour. However, the attempt to encourage him to take control in the above excerpt was plainly too big a step for C. It may have to be shown to him by example first (for example, others in the room take turns to issue directives, and then C has a try). At the same time, reinforcement of his spontaneously occurring directives (such as 'mine'), at least some of the time, will continue to be helpful.

EXERCISE 2.7

Again, think about Carl's understanding of, and response to, the therapist's c-acts.

   Carl and T are still placing balls on sticks. T has picked up a ball.

```
T:  (holds up ball) whose is this one?
C:  (looks at T)
T:  is it yours?
C:  0
T:  yes?
C:  mine (nods, but does not look at T)
```

(0 = zero or non-response)

Comments on Exercise 2.7: Linguistic

Carl appears not to have understood T's questions 'whose is this one?', 'is it yours?'. He does not give a conventional response until the end, when his utterance 'mine' follows a yes/no question where the answer 'yes' or 'no' might have been expected. In view of past usage, C's utterance 'mine' may merely be an expression of frustration and a wish to get on with the game.

Comments on Exercise 2.7: Clinical implications

There are suggestions here that C displays severe limitations in the respondent role. The questions used by T are not only requests for infor-mation, but also perform the role of offering, in this case offering something (the ball) that C clearly wants. He does not seem to understand this, or, if he does, he does not realize that he can obtain the ball by indicating (verbally or non-verbally) that he accepts the offer. Clinically, he will benefit from further modelled role play, this time of offers and accep-tances, along similar lines to that suggested for helping him to produce directives.

EXERCISE 2.8

Think about what is motivating Carl's behaviour (verbal and non-verbal) in this sequence:

Carl, T, Carl's mother (M) and a student observer (A) are taking it in turns to take a formboard piece out of a bag, and place it on to the board. C is finding it very difficult to wait for his turn. We start with C's go.

```
T:  now it must be your go, C
    See what you get
C:  (pulls piece out of bag)
M:  plane
    You like the plane don't you
    Where does the plane go?
C:  (places piece on board)
```

    T: now whose go is it now?
    C: (tries to feel in bag)
    T: I thinks it's A's go
         Shall we give her a go
         (reaches across C with bag)
    A: (chooses a piece and places it on the board)
    T: and now it's Mummy's go
    C: mine (reaches for bag)
    M: Mummy go first
         Mummy's go
         Then yours
         (pulls out piece)
    T: what did Mummy get?
    C: (ignores others, sits with face on table)
    T: whose go is it now?
    C: (reaches in bag)

Comments on Exercise 2.8: Linguistic

Again, C says nothing except 'mine'. Although he responds appropriately (albeit non-verbally) when it is his turn, he seems to understand none of the comments that suggest it is someone else's turn and that he should wait. He tries to continue with the same responses, and, when thwarted, withdraws from the situation.

Comments on Exercise 2.8: Clinical implications

This is a very apt illustration that C has difficulty with the concept of *turn-taking*. Although seen here in the context of a game that involves turns (a popular way of teaching children to wait turns in a relaxed context), it is widely believed that this basic skill is also developed through conversational interaction with others; the child says something, then someone replies, and then it is the child's turn again. Since C only has very limited conversational ability, it is perhaps not surprising that he cannot participate in a turn-taking game. (See Chapter 3 for further discussion of the importance of turn-taking in conversation.)

Summary comments on all clinical examples: linguistic and clinical implications

Looking just at the language used by C in these extracts tells us very little about the nature of his difficulties. The only word he uses with conviction is 'mine', and even this seems to serve a variety of functions: retaining a desirable item, taking a turn in a game, moving an activity back to a routine he understands. Looking at C's communication from the point of view of c-acts, it can be seen that there are severe limitations. He is unable to use language to direct others (except to attract attention), and unable to respond positively to the speech acts of others, such as offers. As a result of these limitations, much of his communication seems negative, showing an apparent unwillingness to cooperate with what is going on. To some extent, this can be correlated with his developmental delay; his inability to see beyond the here and now, his extreme responses when thwarted and his short attention span are all typical of a younger child. However, he also lacks a basic awareness of the potential of communication to achieve desirable goals. He is unable to use communication to influence the behaviour of others, and he seems unable to recognize and respond to suggestions from others that might lead to an enjoyable outcome. At the same time, C is surrounded by adults who have powerful communication skills and who are anxious to use these to extract more acceptable social behaviour from him (his impending entry into nursery school was causing considerable concern). A vicious circle is building up whereby from C's point of view, communication only serves the purpose of thwarting his own wishes. The therapist's role is therefore to motivate C by providing him with successful communicative experiences, while at the same time moving him forward and expanding his repertoire of communicative acts, so that he can participate more fully in what is going on around him. It goes without saying that caregivers need to be guided to follow these principles as well. Until C gains a greater awareness of the power and rewards of successful communication, he is unlikely to be motivated to learn new linguistic skills. Readers wishing to find out more about useful techniques for working with children such as C are referred to the sections on 'naturalistic therapy' approaches in Andersen-Wood and Smith (1997: 72, 85).

Summary

In this chapter we have attempted to look beyond the surface forms of language to what is achieved by the speech act. Speech acts do not show straightforward mapping between form and function, and in indirect speech acts, the illocutionary force of the act does not correspond to the function of the sentence as expressed in grammatical terms (that is, interrogative, imperative, declarative). Many features of the context and participants will be important in interpreting speech acts, and some of the functions of speech acts can be achieved non-verbally, through cries, gesture, facial expression and actions. The term *communicative act* may therefore be more useful. As c-acts can be expressed non-verbally, children begin to develop a repertoire of acts early in life. Subsequent development both enlarges this repertoire and increases the sophistication with which acts are expressed, frequently through a subtle mix of non-verbal behaviour and increasingly complex linguistic structures. This development is dependent on linguistic and cognitive maturation, and on appropriate reinforcement from the environment.

Children may display deficiencies in both the range of acts at their disposal, and the means with which they express them. They may also have difficulties interpreting the c-acts of others. In some more disordered cases, c-acts may be expressed through non-conventional means, and thus run the risk of being ignored or misinterpreted. The speech and language therapist's role will be both to encourage existing communicative behaviour by reinforcement, and to extend the child's repertoire by exposing him or her to models of new behaviour in real communicative contexts.

Chapter 3:
Discourse and
conversational analysis

Key words: discourse, conversational analysis, turn-taking, exchange, topic, interaction.

Aims

In the previous chapter, we looked at how utterances are used communicatively to achieve specific results for the speaker, corresponding to his/her communicative intent. When talking about conversational acts (c-acts) in this way it becomes increasingly difficult to ignore the other participants in the interaction and how they respond. Their response gives some indication as to the success of the original speaker's c-act. At the same time, as will have become clear in Chapter 2, people need to be able to take on the respondent as well as the initiator role in order to communicate successfully. In a longer conversation, or *discourse*, there are further constraints on what is said. Topics of conversation are introduced and terminated in certain conventional ways, as are the conversations themselves. There are generally agreed ways of interrupting, changing the topic and bringing new participants into the conversation.

The study of stretches of language longer than a sentence is referred to as *discourse analysis*. Just as sentences themselves conform to patterns (or grammatical rules), so can discourse be said to do so. Some discourses feature one speaker (or writer) only: lectures or essays are expected to conform to a certain structure in order to be comprehensible to others, and much energy is spent learning to do this and practising the skill. To begin at the end of such a discourse will generally not work, unless this is done for dramatic effect and clearly marked up as such (as may be the case in a novel where the writer begins with a scene from the end of the story, and then proceeds to show the events that lead up to that particular state of affairs). At the same time, the constraints applying to discourse are not as rigid as those that apply to the sentence. Order can be changed for effect, and where there is an unexpected sequence the listener or reader will look for ways to interpret this effectively, where possible making use of their knowledge of the speaker and topic.

The type of discourse we will be dealing with here is spoken and will involve more than one participant. A further type of discourse, that of narrative, is considered in Chapter 5. It has been noted that conversations in this sense also have a recognizable structure; hence the term *conversational analysis (CA)*.

Key questions:
What are the units that go to make up a conversational discourse?
How do initiations and responses relate to one another?
How do initiation–response sequences fit into the wider discourse?
How are conversations managed, in terms of their commencement and ending?
How are topics in conversation identified, introduced and terminated?
How do conversational skills develop in the child?
How may conversations be affected when one of the participants is pragmatically impaired?

Background concepts and issues

Discourse units

In CA, one of the most basic units of analysis is the *exchange*. This is minimally a sequence where one speaker says one thing, to which the other speaker responds. The first speaker's utterance, or *turn*, is referred to as an *initiation*, and the second speaker's turn will constitute a *response*. This suggests, of course, that the exchange can be broken down into smaller units or turns, an exchange consisting minimally of two turns. *Turn-taking* is considered an important skill in children, both in practical terms of being able to take turns to play with a toy (a social skill), or to take a turn in games such as 'Snakes and Ladders', and in terms of being able to take a turn at speaking in a conversation.

Most conversations proceed at a rapid rate, with changeover from speaker to speaker conducted relatively smoothly and fluently. How do people know when it is time to take their turn? Early work by Sacks, Schegloff and Jefferson (1974) identified *transition relevance* points at which it is possible that the conversation will move to another speaker. In some cases these correspond to an obvious 'handing over' – the new speaker has been asked a question, for example – but, in others, the new speaker takes advantage of natural potential break point in the first speaker's utterance, usually corresponding to a sentence, clause or phrase boundary. Speakers use their awareness of prosody, grammatical structure and context to predict when a transition relevance point is coming up. Similarly, the person who is talking will also be able to make such predictions and may forestall a speaker change by indicating through intonation that s/he does not wish to relinquish the turn at this point. Thus, despite the conventions governing conversations, it is still possible for some speakers to dominate. If a speaker interposes a turn at some point other than a transition relevance point, s/he is likely to be perceived as interrupting (although the degree to which interrupting is acceptable varies from culture to culture). It is particularly difficult to find a suitable transition relevance point if one is trying to break into a conversation that is already happening, for instance to report that one of the participants is needed on the telephone.

Speaker turns may be further broken down to individual c-acts. It is possible for a turn to contain more than one c-act, such as when the speaker supplies information in response to a question and then goes on to ask a further question.

Although the exchange is the minimal unit of a conversational discourse, most discourses will feature more than one related exchange. Hoey (1991) looks at the discourse of pairs of foreign language students, practising 'conversation' in a language class. He points out that these interactions lack many of the characteristics of normal conversations, and especially that each exchange stands alone in terms of topic. The next exchange is not related in any way. A typical 'conversation' in this context may look something like this:

A: Hello
B: Hello
A: how are you?
B: very well
A: what did you do last night
B: I went to the film
A: what did you have for breakfast this morning?
B: bacon and eggs
A: do you think priests should be women?
B: not really
A: where are you going to have lunch today?
B: in the café

This conversation looks bizarre because A's questions are totally unrelated to each other. A never picks up and develops one of B's answers further, or asks a related question. Hoey points out that natural conversation is not a skill that needs to be taught to such students, but that they must have the language resources, in particular a large enough vocabulary, to participate in natural conversations in their non-native language. This is important, since it shows that adults with normal mature conversational skills may still encounter difficulties with interaction if their linguistic skills at other levels are limited.

One further odd feature of this hypothetical conversation is that speaker A asks all the questions, whereas speaker B only responds. In a more natural conversation, we would expect speaker B to take over the questioning or *initiating* role at various points. We can predict that in this artificial situation speaker B will later have his 'turn' (used here in a non-conversational-analysis sense) and take on the role of the initiator for a number of conversational turns. One-sidedness of this kind is also a feature of many adult–child interactions, with the adult issuing a series of initiations to which the child gives a minimal response. Where the child is very young s/he may well be unable to maintain a topic beyond one or two exchanges. A further factor will be the interest of the topic to the child; it is frequently suggested that the skill in interacting with children is to find topics of interest to them.

So how does a conversation develop where both participants have adequate language and communication skills? The term *turn* implies just that: a moment when the speaker has the floor. When talking about how a discourse is structured, analysts use the term *move* to describe how speakers move the conversation forward. An exchange of the type already mentioned will consist of an initiating move (which may demand a response), and a responding move from the other participant.

Although conversations will vary in length, and in the number of exchanges devoted to each topic, there will typically be markers both of the beginning and end of whole conversations ('hello, have you got a minute?', 'well, I must go now'), and also of the introduction and closure of topics (for example, 'changing the subject, have you heard from Jim?... ', 'OK, that's fine'). Sinclair and Coulthard (1975), in their seminal study of classroom discourse, identify *frame* and *focus moves*, whereby a teacher will alert the class that a new topic is being introduced (frame) and orientate them regarding the subject matter (focus). Discourse analysts have produced detailed frameworks of the way in which conversation can be structured, and taxonomies of the different types of moves involved (see Stenstrom, 1994 for a recent account, and also the chapter on discourse analysis in Smith and Leinonen, 1992 for a summary). It is important to be aware, however, that although it is possible to identify patterns in the structure of conversations (and also, as we shall see later, that these patterns can be violated), they are essentially fluid. No one decides in advance the exact form and content of the discourse (or if one of the participants attempts to do so, s/he is likely to find her or his attempts blocked by unpredictable contributions from other participants) and it develops according to the influence of the situation, the motivations of participants and what has been said already.

It is, however, possible to identify some patterns as typical of particular situations:

EXERCISE 3.1

Here are two exchanges. Which is the more acceptable and why?

Exchange 1

Speaker A is a teacher, speaker B a pupil.

> A: what is the name of the capital city of France
> B: Paris
> A: Yes, well done.

Exchange 2

Speakers A and B are friends discussing an itinerary.

> A: and then we could go to that port in the South of France, what's it called
> B: Marseilles
> A: Yes, well done.

Comment 3.1

The first thing you may have noted is that each of these exchanges has three parts or moves. Speaker A asks a question (one type of initiation), speaker B answers, or responds, and then speaker A comes back with a comment that somehow evaluates this response. In the classroom situation this seems normal, whereas in a conversation between friends this sort of evaluation feels out of place. The right to evaluate has something to do with the different status of teacher and pupil and with the pedagogic nature of the interaction, and this type of three-part exchange is typical of a teaching situation. Another feature of the classroom situation is that speaker A asks a question to which s/he already knows the answer. This is not a genuine request for information (note that this breaks one of the *felicity conditions* mentioned in Chapter 2; this sort of didactic exchange seems to be appropriate in certain kinds of teaching situations).

The 'evaluative' part of the exchange is often referred to as a *follow-up*. Essentially, it relates to a previous move (in this case, speaker B's response) and does not necessarily have any initiating role. Follow-ups do occur in conversations between equals, but they are often used to indicate that an utterance has been understood, or to express agreement with what has been said.

*   *   *   *   *   *

Studies have been carried out to identify characteristics typical of discourses that take place in socially identifiable situations. An example is the Sinclair and Coulthard study mentioned above, which focuses on the classroom. A further example is a study by Labov and Fanshel (1977), who look at the discourse between analyst and client in psychoanalysis.

Letts (1985a, summarized in 1985b) gives an analysis of the discourse of typical speech and language therapy (SLT) sessions. In this study, she found that SLT discourse could be described using a framework similar to that of Sinclair and Coulthard, and indeed the data contained many characteristics typical of the classroom situation (see also Letts, 1989). In particular, the three-part initiation-response-feedback exchange (the term initiation was replaced by *stimulus* in Letts' model) was found to occur, and therapists used moves specifically to set up and structure activities. Therapy was essentially *structured*, and would nowadays be considered to be 'directive' or 'adult-centred'. It should be noted, however, that the study included a range of patient types and equal numbers of adult and child clients. It is not therefore representative only of therapy with children, although it was noted that the approach to the child clients was more uniform. Perhaps more important is the fact that the data for the study were collected in the early 1980s, and there have been considerable innovations in the delivery of child therapy since then. New approaches that predictably would result in different patterns of therapy discourse include *non-directive therapy*, in which the therapist is far more guided by what the child does (see, for example, Tierney and Cogher, 1994, and also naturalistic therapy as described by Andersen-Wood and Smith, 1997), and an approach to phonological remediation, *Metaphon*, where the child is encouraged to explore and discuss properties of sounds, motivated by his/her own interest and curiosity (Howell and Dean, 1994).

It is interesting to speculate how such approaches might yield different patterns of interaction if looked at using the Letts framework. With non-directive therapy, the three-part exchange is likely to disappear altogether, with the therapist primarily giving feedback in response to initiations from the child (note that feedback in this model is not necessarily concerned with whether something is right or wrong, but includes expansions, extensions of the child's utterances, and agreement). Other utterance types likely to be greater in number are comments from the therapist on the child's actions or about items the child is looking at. The term *information giving* from the original model comes closest to this type of c-act, but was at the time viewed as giving the child information pertinent to the task in hand and therefore still very orientated to the planned adult-directed activity.

Thus, the framework would probably show considerable differences between child-directed and more traditional approaches. With Metaphon, the picture is predicted to be somewhat different, since this remains a highly structured approach. Two possibilities are first, that there would be more role-reversal, as activities take place where the child gives stimuli for the therapist to respond to, and second, that although feedback is given to the child's moves, its content is quite specific. Rather than being corrective in nature, the therapist indicates what he or she has heard by responding 'wrongly' (that is, selecting the 'wrong' picture), and/or by commenting on the properties of the sounds he or she has heard. In the case of Metaphon, therefore, a therapy session might superficially look very similar to the traditional approaches used, but closer inspection is needed of the roles played by child and therapist, and the sort of information that is being exchanged as each takes their turn in the interaction.

We can see, then, how descriptive frameworks for discourse can give insight into the nature of interactions that occur in different social situations. For the child, on the other hand, it is important that an awareness of discourse appropriate to different situations develops, and that s/he has the language skills to be able to conduct a discourse satisfactorily. Even casual and apparently relaxed conversations between friends, talking about nothing in particular, carry important social messages. Very strong claims for such conversations are made by Eggins and Slade (1997):

> casual conversation is a critical linguistic site for the negotiation of such important dimensions of our social identity as gender, generational location, sexuality, social class membership, ethnicity, and subcultural and group affiliations. (Eggins and Slade, 1997: 6)

Plainly, anyone who lacks the skills required here is severely at risk for social isolation.

Exchange sequences

It can be seen from the last section that exchanges consist minimally of an initiation from one speaker followed by a response from another. Sequences of exchanges will be sandwiched between moves that serve to indicate that a topic is being introduced or closed, and whole conversations will be sandwiched between moves that start up or terminate the discourse. As suggested above, some moves merely serve to follow up, or give feedback on, the other speaker's last move. These might be of an evaluative nature (typically in the classroom situation, and also in much

SLT interaction as described by Letts 1985a), or may serve to show that the listener agrees with, or has heard and understood, what has been said. In the latter case, words such as 'yes' and phatic noises such as 'um', 'uhuh' may hardly impinge at all on what the speaker is saying and are sometimes referred to as *back-channelling*. Note that listeners can use back-channelling to indicate that they are listening to a boring discourse, even if they are in fact thinking about something else. Crystal and Davy (1975) point out, though, in the context of second language learning, that use of such 'agreement noises' is also a skilled culturally sensitive activity. Too few or too many, or noises in the wrong place, can give a misleading impression.

The exact course that the sequence of moves takes will, of course, depend on their content, and here the nature of c-acts and their function as moves is crucial. Some c-acts, such as greetings, attention-getters, directives and requests for information are *strongly* initiating, in that a response is clearly expected, whereas others, such as comments, may only require a follow-up of some sort, or require no response at all. One area of great interest to those working with children with pragmatic difficulties is how well they meet the pragmatic expectations of initiating moves. In some cases there may be a failure to respond at all, and in others the response may not be the one that is 'expected', or considered to be *appropriate*. However, there are all sorts of perfectly acceptable reasons why someone might not respond as expected to, for example, a directive or request for information. We shall explore some of these in the following exercise:

EXERCISE 3.2

Can you explain why the responses to these initiations, although not exactly what is expected by the initiation, are acceptable? How, if at all, would you expect the discourse to continue?

(a)
Speaker 1: Will you pick me up from work tonight?
Speaker 2: No, I'm afraid I can't. I'm working late tonight.
(b)
Speaker 1: Are you going to the film tonight?
Speaker 2: What time does it start?
(c)
Speaker 1: Would you mind closing the window?
Speaker 2: Pardon?
(d)
Speaker 1: Are you planning to visit the Monet exhibition?
Speaker 2: Which exhibition?

Comment 3.2

First, you may have noticed that, although all of speaker 1's utterances have an interrogative form, only in (b) and (d) do they have a questioning function, performing the c-act of requesting information. In (a) and (c), speaker 1 is issuing a directive, although (a) could also arguably be a request for information about what speaker 2 will do. In any case, speaker 2 here refuses to comply with the directive (but does supply the requested information) and gives a reason for non-compliance, or excuse. An 'excuse' for non-compliance is an acceptable alternative to responding to a directive, if one does not wish to or is unable to carry out the required action. We would expect the topic to be dropped at this point, or for speaker 1 to suggest why the reason or excuse is not valid (for example, by saying something like: 'that's all right. I'm going to work late too').

In (b), speaker 1's request for information is met by an information request from speaker 2. Speaker 2 plainly needs more information before he can answer the question. We would, however, expect an answer eventually from speaker 2, regarding whether he is going to the film. He could ask a number of further questions – which film it is, who is in it, which cinema it is showing at – but speaker 1 will still eventually expect an answer. What is happening here is that a further question–answer sequence (or further sequences) are 'embedded' in the original sequence. These embedded sequences are sometimes referred to as *side sequences*.

It is sometimes the case, however, that speakers may get so side-tracked by a side sequence that the original initiation becomes somehow lost and is never responded to. There could be a number of reasons for this. Both speakers may become so absorbed by the side sequence that they effectively lose interest in the original initiation. Alternatively, one speaker may be able to give the other speaker the impression that this has happened, or cause the other speaker to forget about the original initiation, because he or she wishes to avoid having to respond to it. This is highly skilled conversational strategy. Finally, speaker 2 may fail to respond to speaker 1's original initiation because s/he is impaired in some way: memory or processing constraints may mean that the original request is forgotten, or, in the case of the pragmatically impaired individual, s/he may simply not be aware of the expectation of a response.

(c) and (d) illustrate two types of *repair* sequences, in both these cases a special type of side sequence. In (c), speaker 2 has failed to hear and/or understand the initiation and demands a straightforward repetition. In (d), one part of the initiation (the name of the exhibition) is not clear, so this part is explicitly queried with a *clarification request*. As with (b), however, the expectation is that eventually the original initiation will be responded to.

Pre-sequences

The competent communicator will sometimes anticipate 'excuses' that a speaker may give when faced with a directive, and use a *pre-sequence* to explore these first. Often this will be a genuine attempt to establish whether the listener can comply with a directive, or accept an invitation, as in the following example:

Speaker 1: Are you busy tonight?
Speaker 2: Not really.
Speaker 1: Well do you fancy going to see a film?
Speaker 2: That's a good idea.

It is, however, a little puzzling that speaker 1 bothers with a pre-sequence here. If speaker 2 is busy, he will merely give this as a reason and decline the invitation. It seems that issues to do with face and politeness are involved here (see Brown and Levinson, 1987). The initiator would like to avoid having a request turned down or an invitation rejected and would therefore prefer not to issue the request or invitation if this is likely to be the case. The pre-sequence allows him to establish this in advance. Note, however, that in the above case, the invitation is still likely to be spoken, as in 'oh, what a shame, I was going to suggest we went to the film'. However, in this case one of the felicity conditions for an invitation does not apply, since speaker A now knows that speaker B is unable to accept. In speech act terms this would no longer function as an invitation.

It is also the case that in many situations people do not like to reject an initiation (in terms of refusing to comply with a request or declining an invitation) unless they can supply a reasonable excuse. Competent communicators can manipulate this when using pre-sequences, so, for example, the conversation above could have developed as follows:

Speaker A: Are you busy this evening?
Speaker B: Not really.
Speaker A: In that case, you can help me clear out the garage.

Note that it is somehow not very acceptable for speaker B to now say that he does not want to clear out the garage; having used up one potential excuse (not being free), he will now have to think of a different one to justify non-compliance. Listeners are, of course, aware of being manipulated in this way, and will often counteract the initiating move in a pre-sequence with a side sequence of their own, beginning something like: 'why are you asking?' Children are also able to use pre-sequences to effect, although these may not be so sophisticated as those used by an adult.

EXERCISE 3:3

In the following example, a formulaic utterance is used to initiate the pre-sequence, which none the less demands a response. What does the child gain here by using this pre-sequence?

> *Child*: D'you know what?
> *Adult*: What?
> *Child*: Well, at school today ... (embarks on long complicated story).

Comment 3:3

This is a strategy commonly used by children. Most adults will feel somehow obliged to respond to the initiation 'd'you know what?' with the question 'what?'. By asking the question, however, the adult is then giving evidence of interest about the event the child wishes to describe, and must then give their full attention to the story that follows. In a world in which a busy adult's attention may be difficult to attract and retain, the child quickly learns this as a good strategy to introduce a topic. Of course, if overused, adults will also learn to counteract the strategy when busy, perhaps by saying something like 'not now, I'm busy' in response to the child's opening question. Older children and adults will have more sophisticated means of introducing a story of this kind, with utterances such as 'something really interesting happened to me today. Shall I tell you about it?'.

*   *   *   *   *   *

'Appropriate' responses

As we have seen above, responses to initiations can be perfectly acceptable without being the obvious expected ones. If an unexpected response occurs in a conversation, the participants will work with the assumption that the response is intended to be relevant and appropriate (see Chapter 7). If it does not immediately make sense as a response, the listener will work hard to try to make it make sense.

EXERCISE 3.4

The following are all uttered by speaker B in response to the request for information from speaker A: 'where's the tea-towel gone?' Can you construct a situation for each where they are relevant and meaningful responses? Are there any for which this is impossible?

(1) Into the washing machine
(2) Just leave them to drain
(3) Where's what?
(4) What tea-towel?
(5) Ten green bottles
(6) Why ask me?
(7) Friday
(8) Did you want to dry the dishes?
(9) Is it my birthday?
(10) Yes

Comment 3.4

(1) is a straightforward response to the question, giving the location of the tea-towel. Note that it could be perceived as a not particularly helpful response, since it may not be possible to retrieve the tea-towel from this location. If speaker A was in fact intending to use a tea-towel, then a more helpful response might suggest in addition where more tea-towels can be found ('look in that drawer'). Many of the remaining responses given actually assume that the initiation 'where's the tea-towel gone?' is functioning as an *offer* (to dry dishes) as well as a request for information. Response (8) queries this interpretation explicitly.

Responses (2) and (9) actually respond to an implicit offer, rather than the more explicit request for information. In (2) speaker B declines the offer, suggesting an alternative solution (at which point the interaction about the tea-towel may well finish), and we can interpret (9) as a potentially sarcastic expression of surprise that the offer has been made. (9) apparently shows that speaker B is searching for a reason for the offer being made. Subsequently, we might expect the offer to be accepted.

(3), (4) and (6) are all ostensibly requests for repair, querying what is being asked for (3), the existence of the thing being asked for (4), and the justification for asking speaker B in the first place (6). Note that all of these requests for clarification could be posed with a degree of sarcasm in a situation where speaker A rarely dries dishes. (4) and (6) are also querying the felicity conditions for speaker A's request, specifically whether s/he has reason to believe that what is being asked for actually exists (4), or whether speaker B can reasonably be expected to know the answer (6).

This leaves the much more problematical responses (5), 'ten green bottles', (7), 'Friday', and (10) 'yes'. At first glance they do not seem to relate to the initiation in any way, be it as a request for information or as an offer. We might be tempted to say that these responses are disordered. However, by applying enough ingenuity it may be possible to construct scenarios where such responses are acceptable and informative. Response (5) may refer to a location that has been idiosyncratically christened 'ten green bottles' by the participants, perhaps because green bottles are stored there. (7) may be a reference to an event that regularly occurs on a Friday (the collecting of tea-towels to be laundered, for example). Finally, 'yes' (depending on intonation used) may be an abbreviated form for something like: 'yes, that's a good question. It's really puzzling, what happens to all the tea-towels round here'. This brings us to a problem that will be discussed further when inappropriacy and disordered discourse are considered. If the analyst looks at some sort of record of the discourse, s/he is unable to know exactly the state of knowledge and motives of the speakers at the time. Different analysts may interpret moves in different ways (this was also discussed in Chapter 2 with reference to c-acts), and may well disagree about whether a response is appropriate or not. Detailed notes on context and intonation patterns used are obviously essential, but, even then, the true situation can only be inferred.

Developmental notes

Much of the work on the early development of discourse focuses on the role played by adults when interacting with very young children. We have already seen in Chapter 2 how adults will attribute communicative intent to a baby's vocalizations, even in the absence of any evidence of attempt to communicate. This behaviour fulfils the valuable function of showing the child the potential of communicative behaviour to achieve goals such as food, comfort and adult attention.

In addition, adults will work hard with infants to set up discourse sequences. As the child starts to explore the use of language and add this to his/her communicative repertoire of vocalizations, facial expressions and gestures, the adult will aim to build on and extend the child's attempts in various ways. Initiations from the child may be followed by comments and further initiations from the adult on the same topic. The adult will also initiate exchanges by drawing the child's attention to things in the environment that may be of interest to him or her, and responding and initiating further when the child responds. What is evident at this early stage is that the adult takes all the responsibility for setting up and pursuing the discourse (see McLaughlin, 1998).

It is clear that, in addition to providing the child with information about how discourse is structured and how it can be applied to various ends, the adult's ability to set up a discourse with the child also permits valuable lessons to be learned about language itself. For example, Harris (1992) compared the interaction of mothers of a group of children acquiring language relatively quickly, with that of mothers of children who were slower (note, however, that all of these children were considered to have language developing within normal limits). She found that the mothers of the faster group commented on and named items as the child was attending to them. Less successful interactions seemed to be the result of a timing mismatch between the child's attending to an item, and the mother's comment on it. There is a wide literature, beginning with the seminal collection of papers edited by Snow and Ferguson (1977), on the characteristics of parent–child interaction and the ways in which this may work to enhance the child's language development. Wells (1985) shows how particular features of parental input seem to support the child's language acquisition. Attempts have been made to apply this sort of approach to parental advice programmes for cases of language delay or disorder (see, for example, Clezy, 1979; the Hanen programme (Fryer, 1994); and Ward, 1999). Caution should be exercised here for a number of reasons. First, it has been shown that adult–child interaction can vary considerably across cultures (for example, Goody, 1978; Schieffelin, 1979). Schieffelin noted that the Kaluli people 'teach' interactive roles, and therefore presumably discourse skills, through getting children to imitate, something that is not reported in the literature on American or European children. A second consideration is that the development of discourse is a two-way process, with the child sooner or later having to play his or her part in initiating and sustaining discourse. Wells points out that the normal children in his study 'appeared to differ in their willingness to engage in interaction' (Wells, 1985: 416). The impact on adult–child interaction of the child being an inadequate or unwilling communicator also needs to be addressed. As was discussed in Chapter 2, the effective use of c-acts by the child involves the ongoing development of several different types of ability – cognitive, social and linguistic. Where any of these is impaired in some way, further modifications to input are likely to be required in order to best help the child, as well as more targeted remediation to help the child overcome deficits where possible. Finally, Conti-Ramsden and Dykins (1991) found consistent styles of interaction in families containing one language impaired and one language-normal child at the same linguistic stage. This suggests that style of interaction is not a causative factor (at least not for these families) for language impairment, and that modifying interaction will not necessarily have any direct benefit.

Another aspect of early adult–child interaction that is frequently mentioned is the use of ritualized repetitive games, such as 'peekaboo'. The child increasingly plays an interactive role in these sequences and learns to anticipate the next move. It is thought that the highly ritualized nature of these games allows the child to explore and develop their discourse features, without having to focus too much on linguistic content. For example, Dewart and Summers (1995) mention this sort of activity under the development of interaction and conversation, in the 'birth to nine months' phase (p.8).

Conversational development beyond the infant stage is characterized by increasing participation in ongoing discourse, by the ability to cope with longer discourses, and by increasing sophistication in using devices to introduce topics, maintain topics and to pursue argument and discussion. Both McTear (1985a) and Dewart and Summers (1995) also indicate that discourse further develops through play, either playing with linguistic forms, or conducting 'pretend' conversations in which certain roles are sustained. The child has this further avenue for developing his/her interactional skills, in addition to the experience of successful interaction with others.

Dewart and Summers (1995) note that children begin to initiate interactions through non-verbal means (pointing, vocalizations) in the 9–18 month period, and begin to use speech in conversations, initially to respond to verbal stimuli, after 18 months. The child will also make attempts to respond to 'repair' requests from adults, either by repeating or revising an utterance. S/he may initiate conversations through using vocatives as attention getters, and after age 3 years can use more sophisticated strategies of the 'do you know what?...' type. At this point, children will also start to construct 'pretend' conversations. After 4 years of age, the normally developing child is able to request repairs, and is becoming able to adapt to conversational partners who may differ with regard to features such as age and familiarity. Timing of turns and attempts to join conversations become more precise and the child can initiate and terminate conversations. Crucially, throughout this period of development, the child has been able to sustain participation in longer and longer sequences of turns.

McTear's (1985a) study of the interaction between two girls between the ages of about 4 and 6 years gives further insight into the development of conversational skills. Many of the basic interactional skills were in place before this study commenced. For example, the girls were able to initiate and respond appropriately, to reinitiate where necessary, and to request and make repairs. They also displayed a strong awareness of the structure of turns. Where overlaps inevitably occurred, one would stop, and the other would frequently repeat the 'overlap' part of her utterance so that it did not get lost. As suggested by Dewart and Summers (1995), exchange sequences between the two children increased in length, but also in complexity. Simple initiation–response sequences were increasingly replaced by sequences where utterances both responded to the previous utterance and initiated a further response (McTear's R/I moves). Turns also developed in the sense of including more than one related act, such as including both a request and a justification for the request. Disputes were particularly interesting in this respect, beginning in the early recordings as repetitive sequences of assertion and counter-assertion, and developing into more complex arguments involving justifications and challenges of previous assertions. McTear also provides some interesting illustrations of how intonation patterns enter into the dialogue and have a mirroring effect, especially with verbal play sequences. From the point of view of contributing linguistic skills, McTear notes the increasingly sophisticated use of discourse connectors (for example, 'well', 'anyway', 'otherwise'), and the importance of grammatical skill in making a successful initiation (or reinitiation) about objects or persons outside the immediate physical context (see Chapter 4, on referring expressions).

When it comes to later conversational development, McTear points out that this is difficult to observe in the same naturalistic way, partly because children will become more conscious of being observed, and partly because the range of contexts in which children have to learn to interact effectively becomes vastly greater. One of these contexts is, of course, school, and there is evidence that some children may find this new environment a difficult one in which to use previously acquired conversational skill. McTear cites a study by Wells and Montgomery (1981) where a child called Rosie shows only very limited ability when a teacher attempts to interact (on a one-to-one basis) with her, despite showing much greater conversational skill when she is more engaged by the topic. At the same time, we know from the work of Sinclair and Coulthard (1975) that interactions in school tend to be much more tightly structured than those at home, at least as far as teaching to a group is concerned. Tizard and Hughes (1984), in their study of young working-class and middle-class girls talking at home and at school, noted a discrepancy between the two environments for the working-class children. The girls did not display the language ability that they clearly possessed when interacting with teachers in the school environment. The teachers, having a different style of interaction from the girls' mothers, were not able to facilitate longer or more complex sequences of talk. It is possible that difficulties in adapting to different norms of interaction were inhibiting the children here.

As with Chapter 2, the reader is referred to McTear and Conti-Ramsden (1992) and Andersen-Wood and Smith (1997) for overviews of conversational development.

Conversational impairment

When discussing the difficulties of carrying out research on development of conversational skills in older children, McTear states that 'there is no model of the skilled adult conversationalist which might inform such work' (McTear, 1985a: 201). This lack of a clear adult normative model is also a problem when it comes to looking at impairment. Although gross abnormalities of interaction are easily recognizable, in some cases problems may blend into the less proficient end of normal. Studies of impaired individuals have typically tried to identify pragmatic errors, or 'inappropriacy', occurring within a discourse (see Chapter 1). It is important to recognize that conversational errors occur in perfectly normal conversations, and may or may not be subject to repair processes. (This will probably depend on the communicative importance to the participants of the 'breakdown'. An utterance that is merely a throwaway remark may pass unchallenged if not heard properly or entirely understood. Repair will be requested where the information in the utterance is of potential value to the listener.) As already suggested, listeners can very often construe a possible logical interpretation for a strange utterance, by creating a context in which it could be uttered appropriately. In fact, this seems to be something we prefer to do if possible, rather than run the risk of a total breakdown of the conversation. Thus, it may be that other participants collude with those with conversational impairment to give an impression of a smooth-running conversation (but leave the interaction unsure of what they have been talking about). Such collusion needs to be distinguished from facilitating interaction; since the impaired participant is unaware that the interaction has been unsatisfactory, a collusion approach can be less than helpful.

Ultimately, judgements of conversational impairment seem to reflect the proportion of utterances that are strange; one or two in a discourse may be the result of minor misunderstandings, and more may suggest a real problem. It is, however, possible to see how interactions fail to get started or to progress because of some flaw in the approach taken by one of the interactants. An early case study by McTear (1985b) of a boy with conversational disability showed how he seemed to find it difficult to move the conversation forward by providing any more than minimal responses to initiations. Furthermore, where there was a lull in the conversation, the boy would fill it by repeating all or part of his previous utterance, rather than beginning a new initiation. The problems displayed by the two children in the Willcox and Mogford-Bevan (1995) study have already been mentioned in Chapter 2. Nigel, one of the boys, fails to follow up attention-getting devices. So, although he may successfully attract someone's attention, the conversation cannot progress further. On other occasions, he fails to signal at all to an addressee that he is initiating an interaction, or may use a declarative form to initiate that only weakly demands a response. The outcome is that there may be attempts to start a discourse, but these fail early on.

Another area in which children with conversational impairment may display difficulty is in 'slotting in' appropriately to a discourse that has been set up by a conversational partner. This may be seen particularly in adult–child discourse in educational or remedial contexts, where the adult will have a particular agenda, or planned activity, that they wish to follow. Typically, this may happen when the activity is at too high a level for the child.

EXERCISE 3.5

The following examples come from data that are reported more fully in Letts and Reid (1994). Can you decide first, what was the intention of the adult in setting up these interactions, and second, how these intentions are disrupted by the child's contributions?

(A = Adult, C = child)

(1)
A is showing C a picture-card sequence featuring a cat and a fish:
A: so look
    the fish is in the bowl
    and the cat comes
C: I can eat paper you know
A: you found some paper, haven't you

(2)
A: I'm going to show you some pictures and you have to guess the last part
    these children have lots of pets
    the turtle is hers, the budgie is his, and the dog is (*deliberately left unfinished*)
C: hers
A: every day when John gets sleepy (*deliberately left unfinished*)
C: everyday he gets sleep (*tries to develop story further*)

Comment 3.5

In (1), the adult is beginning to tell the story, and we can guess that at some point the story will be handed over to the child to tell, as an exercise in narrative. However, the child interrupts with an unrelated statement. This may also be a violation of turn-taking conventions, but even if the adult was willing to concede the turn at that point, the child abruptly changes the topic in a way that in some circumstances would be considered inappropriate (note, however, that this is followed up by the adult, rather than the adult attempting to revert immediately to the story). In this particular instance, the child may have been bored with the topic/activity, rather than the problem being that of the level being too high; in fact, the level may have been pitched too low.

In (2) the child is set a task to do, to 'finish' the sentence. It is certainly arguable that the nature of the task is not made clear by the adult, who just refers to 'guessing the last part'. The child manages to complete one sentence successfully, but then with the next item repeats the whole sentence and takes the discourse off in some creative direction of his own. This task is, of course, highly artificial; however, the child might be expected to recognize this sort of discourse from previous experience of the remediation context.

For both (1) and (2) it is impossible to know whether the child has deliberately disrupted the discourse because the task is tedious (displaying pragmatic skill), whether this is a natural response to a task that is too difficult, or whether the child does not understand the discourse conventions that apply here.

*   *   *   *   *   *

Despite these observations, however, it is apparent that gross violations of conversational rules may not be a defining characteristic in pragmatic impairment. Adams and Bishop (1989) looked at four aspects of conversational discourse – exchange structure, turn-taking, repairs and cohesion (see Chapter 4) – in 57 children with specific language impairment (SLI), of which a subgroup of 14 were said to fit the description of semantic-pragmatic disorder (SPD). It was noted that the SPD children produced more initiations than other children (both SLI and normal controls), and that some of them violated turn-taking conventions with excessive interruptions. However, Adams and Bishop state in their discussion that 'our impression ... was that analysis of these aspects of conversational behaviour did not capture the essence of what was abnormal about the language of children with semantic-pragmatic disorder' (Adams and Bishop 1989: 238). They go on to suggest that an effort to define which features lead to an impression of conversational inappropriacy would be more useful.

These 'inappropriate' conversational behaviours have more to do with the content and length of turns than the overall structure of the discourse. In a subsequent study of the same group of children, Bishop and Adams (1989) identify the following as typical of the SPD group: supplying both too little and too much information to a conversational partner, and unusual or socially inappropriate content or style, in addition to problems with expressive syntax and semantics. The features considered under unusual or socially inappropriate content and style, however, do include topic drift and unmarked topic shift, suggesting that the children are unaware of conventional ways of shifting or changing the topic of a conversation. They also include inappropriate questioning in the sense that the adult could not possibly know the answer, or the child already knew the answer. As discussed in Chapter 2, these questions violate felicity conditions for 'information seeking', and are associated with the behaviour of much younger children.

The Pragmatics/Discourse Coding System is described in Letts and Reid (1994). This is based on conversational data collected from four children attending a special school for children with severe language impairment, who were considered by their speech-language therapists and teachers to have problems of a semantic-pragmatic nature. Features that seem to violate discourse conventions (in addition to those mentioned in Exercise 3.5 above) are as follows:

1. *Complete topic shift*: the child's next utterance after an initiation from the other participant in the conversation does not relate in any way to the initiation.
2. *Tangential response*: the child's next utterance after an initiation is not entirely unrelated, but seems to go off 'at a tangent'.
3. *Use of side sequence*: the child starts a side sequence in response to an initiation, but never gets back to responding to the original initiation.

There is, then, some evidence that children with pragmatic problems show evidence of conversational impairment. One explanation for these difficulties is an inability to set any individual utterance within the wider context of the ongoing discourse (see Chapter 6 on pragmatic compre-hension for further discussion). This impression is confirmed in a recent study by Bishop (1998) using her *Children's Communication Checklist* (CCC). One of the subscales of the checklist that is reported to distinguish between SLI and SPD children, is given the heading 'use of conversational context'. Some of the child's immediate responses to initiations may be perfectly appropriate; others may cease to be appropriate once the wider context is taken into account. (Incidentally, Bishop notes in this paper that the term pragmatic language impairment (PLI) may be preferable to semantic-pragmatic disorder (SPD), as little evidence of semantic difficulty has been found for these children. See also Chapter 1.)

Inter-rater reliability

In the above discussion of conversational disorder, *appropriateness* was a term used on several occasions. In looking at a conversation, judgements are made about the appropriateness of an utterance in terms of how it fits into the structure of the conversation (see also Chapter 1). There are a number of factors that render these judgements difficult to make, including the following:

- Without having been a participant, it is not always possible to assess what is appropriate in a particular context; there may be contextual factors that the analyst is unaware of.
- People will differ in terms of what they perceive as inappropriate; it is not possible to apply hard and fast rules as it is with, for example, grammatical errors.
- Even where an utterance is perceived as inappropriate by other participants in the conversation, there may be reasons apparent only to the speaker which would render it appropriate. The child may have experience of, or feelings about, the subject matter of the conversation, which are not known to the other participants. Additionally (and very important in the context of language impaired children), the child may have misunderstood or been slow to process what has gone before, or his or her own contributions may have been misinterpreted. Participants in the conversation may be effectively 'speaking at cross-purposes' as a result.

Leinonen and Smith (1994) show that when asked to rate utterances as inappropriate or not, raters may be influenced by their own training and background, particularly with regard to whether they consider inappropriacy to be the result of adult or child utterances in an adult–child interaction. As a consequence of all these factors, when carrying out research in this area, it is important to try to get as high a degree of inter-rater reliability as possible, both with regard to identifying instances of 'inappropriacy' and in classifying these instances if some sort of classification system is used. Letts (1991) discusses reliability measures for the Bishop and Adams (1989) study, and the Letts and Reid (1994) study discussed above. Bishop and Adams, using a correlation approach, obtained correlations between 0.688 and 0.874, for identifying instances of inappropriacy. Correlations for categories of inappropriacy varied considerably according to category, from very low to very high (that is, above 0.9), depending on the category (especially good results applied to the categories of 'too much information', 'violation of exchange structure' and 'unusual content/use'). For the Pragmatics/Discourse Coding System (Letts and Reid, 1994), an item-by-item approach was used, applied only to the categorization of already identified instances of inappropriacy. Agreement between raters ranged from about 60% to 85%. We would suggest that, to be of any value, inter-rater reliability for analysis of research data in this area needs to be about 80%, and, even then, 20% of the data will be unreliably classified. When using categorization systems of this type as a clinical tool, the problem is not so serious (since the clinician will be looking for general indications of where the child's conversational difficulties seem to lie), providing that any reassessment carried out to evaluate change is conducted by the same individual.

Clinical data

EXERCISE 3.6

P is a 7-year-old child who is reported to have 'autistic tendencies'. At times he makes grunting noises which are not readily interpretable by the listener, but could indicate anxiety in this situation. The excerpt given below is part of an assessment session, where the therapist (T) is trying to ascertain and demonstrate P's problems, rather than provide remediation (although, of course, future remediation may be planned on the basis of these findings). It should be noted however that P was not really an appropriate referral to this particular assessment clinic, where the focus is mainly on linguistic skills. This factor probably exacerbated the unsatisfactory nature of the interaction between P and T. She is trying to start off with a game of 'pair-it' lotto (picture cards have to be matched up with pictures of items from the same semantic field). Several people are in an adjoining room, watching the session on closed circuit video, and the session is also being video-recorded. P cannot see these observers, but is aware that there are people in the adjoining room. As the excerpt begins, P has just picked up a toy clown.

Your task is to pick out 'problem points' in the discourse. You should focus particularly on turn-taking, responses to initiations and the way in which topics are introduced and terminated (by both T and P).

(X = unintelligible syllable, * = utterances overlap, . = short pause, 0 = zero response, ? is used where the question seems to be genuine. Where T uses rising intonation with an unfinished sentence, she is prompting P to supply the missing part of the sentence)

1. T: perhaps he (*the clown*) can watch us play the game
       what's he doing?
2. P: what's this toy for?
3. T: oh, it's just for playing with
4. P: can I throw
5. T: well if you put him here
       then he can watch us *play the game
6. P: *XX play
       (*makes noises*)

7.	T:	where do we see clowns?
8.	P:	in the. is there a laughing clown as well?
9.	T:	um I don't think there is a laughing clown
		no
		I think we've only got one clown
10.	P:	(*makes noises*)
11.	T:	I think we might have some more pictures here, P
		are you going to come and have a look
		or are you going to have a look at a picture
12.	P:	I'm going to go through the telescope (*peers through front of wall-mounted camera*)
13.	T:	I don't think you can see anything through there
14.	P:	what's that called?
15.	T:	they're just picture books
		you come and have a look here
		and I'll show you *what these pictures are
16.	P:	*I'm going to throw
17.	T:	what are you going to throw?
		hm?
		you come and *look at these X
18.	P:	*can we have the next door? (*insistent intonation*)
19.	T:	P, if you come and *sit down
20.	P:	*can we be at the next door thing? (*insistent intonation*)
21.	T:	yes
		afterwards you can go next door
		and you can see yourself on television later
		(*returning to game*) so we're going to take it in turns, P
22.	P:	when I was at home
		would you see me on telly?
23.	T:	not at home
		just here
		but we can do that later, if you do all your work first
24.	P:	not finished?
25.	T:	no, we haven't finished yet because we've got to play this game
26.	P:	(*expletive*)
27.	T:	well what we've got to do
		we're going to turn this card over *and we're
28.	P:	*that's my hand (*points to 'hand' on picture lotto card*)
29.	T:	that's right
		and we've got to see which one it goes with
		which one do you think it goes with?
30.	P:	there (*points to correct picture on large card – 'glove'*)
31.	T:	that's right
		the hand goes with the (*rising intonation*)
32.	P:	there
33.	T:	the glove
		'cos we put a hand inside the glove
		it's my turn now
34.	P:	(*points*) that's the cotton

35. T: (*picking up card*) hm
        I've got a spaceman and it goes with the rocket
36. P: XX playing a game first
        (*reaches across to T's pile of lotto cards*)
37. T: hm
        that's your pile (*moves P's hand over to his own pile*)
        turn one of yours over
38. P: this is cotton (*has in fact picked up a 'letter'*)
39. T: what's that one
40. P: a letter
        for the cotton
41. T: for the cotton (*laughs*)
42. P: (*laughs*)
43. T: no
        where does the letter go
44. P: for the cooker (*places letter on 'cooker' picture*)
45. T: for the cooker
        *no
46. P: *no
47. T: what does the letter go with, P
        (*comments as P tries various inappropriate pictures*)
        not the rabbit hutch
        no
        not the cat
        which one does it go with?
48. P: with the cat (*laughs*)
49. T: no, it doesn't
        which one does it go with, P
        look carefully
        which one do you think
50. P: must not say (*expletive*)
51. T: which one do you think the letter goes with, *P
52. P: (*expletive*)
        yes (*looks abruptly up at T*)
53. T: goes with the (*rising intonation*)
54. P: must not say (*expletive*)
55. T: goes with the letterbox doesn't it
56. P: where's my drink?
57. T: you've already had one, haven't you
58. P: what flavour was it
59. T: you tell me *what flavour it was
60. P: *do some people have a meal at the pub and cafés?
61. T: some people do, don't they
62. P: do they have sausage rolls on toast?
63. T: um, not usually on toast
64. P: do they have beans on toast?
65. T: hm
        beans on toast, yes
66. P: who likes beans on toast

67. T: I don't know
              do you?

68. P: 0

69. T: do you like beans on toast?

70. P: 0

71. T: hm
              I do sometimes
              look at mine, P (*picks up lotto card*)
              I've got a brush and it goes with the dustpan
              your turn
              you turn one over (*turns card over for P*)
              see what you've got

72. P: (*points*) what's that called?

73. T: a screwdriver
              now what have you got
              some (*rising intonation*)

74. P: foxes (*picture is in fact of 'kittens'*)

75. T: are they foxes

76. P: (*laughs*)

77. T: what are they
              they're baby (*rising intonation*)

78. P: bears

79. T: baby bears?

80. P: no

81. T: what are they

82. P: baby foxes

83. T: they go like this
              miaow

84. P: (*imitates miaow sound*)

85. T: so what are they

86. P: cats

87. T: baby cats
              So where do they go
              *they go (*rising intonation*)

88. P: *(*expletive*)

89. T: where do they go, P (*puts card into his hand*)

90. P: (*noises*)

91. T: look, P
              look
              look at the card

92. P: (*looking away*) are those from school? (*points*)

93. T: hm

94. P: from school?

95. T: no
              look
              with Mummy cat
              you put them with Mummy cat because they're baby kittens and
              they go with Mummy cat
              my turn

               *I've got a screwdriver
96. P: *(*noises, gets up from chair*)
               babies do that
97. T: do they
98. P: (*makes noises – continuing over what T is saying*)
99. T: they cry, don't they
               babies cry
               what are you looking at over there?

Comment 3.6

P shows evidence of problems in all the areas mentioned above. First, there are numerous instances of interruptions of the adult's turn, generally not at the sort of syntactic boundaries that might be appropriate transition relevance points (for example, 5/6, 15/16, 27/28). P also fails to respond to T's initiation on several occasions, either by producing an unrelated initiation of his own (2, 8, 54, 92) or by not responding verbally at all (68, 70, both cases where a 'gap' was left by the adult in the interaction for P to answer her question). Finally, P changes the topic abruptly, with no sense of any marker of topic shift being required (12, 56, 60). You might also note that he violates felicity conditions with some of his questions (for example, 58 – he presumably knows the flavour of the drink he has just consumed, and so should not need to ask. In 66, he asks a question to which the adult, in this context, could not be expected to know the answer).

    T tries hard to maintain P's involvement in the topic of her choice (the picture lotto game), with limited success. She follows up some of P's spontaneous initiations (for example, his question about meals in pubs and cafés, line 60, and his subsequent questions about food), but others she largely ignores (for example, line 14, his query about what something is called; line 18, his first request to go next door). While these items are responded to, T does not follow up the topic, but tries to bring the topic back to the planned activity. Some of P's utterances do not seem to be designed to elicit a response, but are more 'speech to himself' (for example, line 16: 'I'm going to throw', line 50: 'must not say'). This is discussed further under clinical interpretation below.

    On the other hand, there are instances where P manages to sustain stretches of coherent discourse. In 20, he asks to go next door and tries to follow up T's comment on the television by asking whether this will happen at home (22). He then asks for clarification following T's comment that he must do his work first, with the query 'not finished?' (24). A rather similar sequence occurs in turns 60–66, where P starts with a question, and then follows up T's answer with related questions. In turns 39–48, although P does not grasp how he is supposed to match up the pictures, he goes through a sequence of trying various options and laughing with T at his mistakes (in fact, this seems to be an attempt to 'cover up' his lack of knowledge and pretend that he knows the answer really and is just joking; it could be argued that this is quite a clever pragmatic strategy!).

Linguistic interpretation

During this session P speaks clearly and there are few instances of unintelligibility. Phonology is normal. Syntax also seems to be normal, as far as one can tell from the extract. P makes no grammatical errors, and although there are no complex sentences in this sample, he is able to form questions accurately (see, for example, turns 2, 60, 66). There is some evidence that sequence of tenses may be a problem for him. In turn 22, P appears to be asking something like 'when I go home, will you be able to see me on the telly?', but he uses the past tense form of the verb *to be* – 'when I was at home', followed by a conditional – 'would you see me?'. This may relate to some of the semantic problems that are also apparent in these data, the time aspect of tense relations being something he is unclear about.

P's use of lexical items shows evidence of potential semantic confusions. He fails to access the words *kittens* or *cats* in turn 74, and instead uses a semantically related word, *foxes*. When challenged, he changes this to a further type of furry animal, *bears* (however, it is possible that the picture is not as helpful as it could be at this point). There is evidence that P's vocabulary is impoverished. He avoids naming the item *glove* (turn 32) and when he picks up the *letter* picture, he perseverates with *cotton* that he has identified earlier (turn 38). An awareness of not knowing the words for things may be apparent in his frequent requests for the names of things (for example, turns 14, 72), reminiscent of a very much younger child. These requests may also, of course, reflect his current developmental level of vocabulary acquisition. Finally, P is unable to actually understand the game being played, which is dependent (or is assumed to be dependent) on an awareness of how things are related to one another in meaning. This is made very clear when he says that the *letter* is 'for the cotton' (40), something clearly unrelated, and then goes on to try to match the letter with other unrelated pictures. Of course, this sort of ability is also dependent on cognitive skills, and we might wonder how cognitively delayed P is.

There is evidence that, at a syntactic level, he knows the sort of response that might be required for particular questions. In 8, he begins to respond to T's *where* question with a prepositional phrase 'in the', which would give a location. However, for whatever reason, he fails to complete this utterance and moves on to an unrelated initiation. This seems to reflect an awareness at the syntactic level – that is, that *where* questions are generally responded to with a prepositional phrase.

It is at the level of discourse, however, that P's problems are most striking. His interruptions of turns, his difficulties responding to initiations from others and his abrupt shift of topic, all suggest a lack of awareness of how language works in conversations. These are all suggestive of a very much younger child.

Clinical interpretation

A child such as P presents the clinician with some immediate serious questions. His interactive skills are plainly nowhere near what one would expect from a 7 year old. In addition, his non-verbal behaviour is bizarre – something that is not brought out in the transcript given above. As well as the grunting noises already mentioned, P avoids eye contact and is frequently distracted and stares around the room (this happens just prior to his 'yes' in turn 52; P gazes around the room, utters an expletive, and then turns abruptly to T as if aware that she has said something that he has not heard). Furthermore, his posture and movements are awkward and somewhat bizarre. One aspect of his verbal behaviour that we have not commented on above is P's use of stereotyped utterances, in this case an expletive. It could be argued that he uses this when being pushed to produce a response he is incapable of (it would be interesting to look at more data and see whether this sort of pattern emerges). Intuitively, it seems unlikely that he fully appreciates the social meaning carried by an expletive, and he is certainly not aware of appropriate situations in which to use it. It is also apparent that he is aware that he is not supposed to use it, as in turn 50 he says 'must not say (*expletive*)'. Here he is using language to regulate his behaviour, something again that is characteristic of much younger children, who have not yet managed to 'internalize' such regulative comments.

From the transcribed data given here it is difficult to judge whether P's communicative behaviour represents his developmental level, or whether there is something unusual or deviant about it. Many behaviours are typical of a very much younger child, notably his interruptions of the other's turns, his abrupt changes of topic, his violation of felicity conditions for questions and his attempts to regulate his own behaviour through verbalization. What perhaps gives an overwhelming picture of oddity is the mismatch of these behaviours with some of the more positive behaviours mentioned in the comment after the exercise – the ability to sustain a sequence of turns about where people go to eat (not in the 'here and now') and the sequence where he tries various options on the board, and perhaps more particularly, his relatively advanced linguistic skills in terms of phonology and syntax. This illustrates a recurring problem with the delay/deviance dichotomy. It is often possible to find examples of the most unexpected behaviour in 'normal' development, especially if one goes back far enough, but such behaviours will often seem bizarre in the context of the much older child.

However, when P's non-verbal behaviour is also taken into account, things start to look much less normal. Here he shows problems that clearly are not purely of a developmental nature. Many of P's behaviours, verbal and non-verbal, are suggestive of autism, and indeed P has already been described as having 'autistic tendencies'. The clinician would need to seek further information from a psychologist, paediatrician or child psychiatrist regarding P's non-verbal cognitive skills, and the possible diagnosis. Any intervention would need to be planned in the context of knowledge about these aspects. From what little is known of P so far, the following might be two areas that would benefit from attention:

1. *Basic interactive skills*: P is willing to interact with those around him, but does not benefit from rewarding interactions because of his current difficulties. Interactions need to be rewarding for him, and in order to ease the situation he needs to learn to respect turntaking conventions and that the initiations of others, as well as his own initiations, merit a relevant response. Again, the source of his problems in these areas would need to be taken into consideration. If he fails to participate because he does not understand what is going on, then interactions must be geared to his developmental social and cognitive level. If his interactive behaviour is mainly the result of the social difficulties that are part of autism, then interaction work would need to take into account some of the special difficulties autistic individuals have in relating to and communicating with others. In reality, it may be the case that P's difficulties with interaction stem from more than one source, and remediation would need to be planned accordingly. Whatever the true position may be, it is plain that P is unaware of the rewarding nature of interactions with others, and has only made shaky progress with the early stages of discourse development. For more information on appropriate remediation, see Andersen-Wood and Smith (1997) and Jordan and Powell (1995).

2. *Attention work*: P is unable to remain focused on an interaction or activity for any length of time and is easily distracted. This could be a primary problem, or could be a feature of the activity being too difficult for him. This would warrant further investigation. His easy distractibility fits with stage 1 of Cooper, Moodley and Reynell's (1978) attention levels, but he does show that he can focus on a topic for at least a short length of time. The problem seems to be more one

of discriminating what to focus on. Instead of screening out some stimuli in favour of, for example, spoken language, he seems equally drawn to any of the items around the room and even to distractions of his own making, such as the noises he is making. Judgements should not be made, however, on the basis of this one excerpt, since P's poor attention may be result of boredom or anxiety. Further observation over time is required.

Summary

It is possible to identify certain patterns in spoken conversations, plus some conventions that people follow, and frameworks have been developed to describe the structure of such discourses. Some discourse settings, such as the classroom, have specific characteristics, and we have seen how descriptive frameworks for discourse can be used to identify these.

Through their experience of personal relationships, children develop the ability to conduct longer and more sophisticated conversations gradually throughout the pre-school years and beyond. At the same time, their widening social world brings them into an increasing range of contexts where different discourse norms will apply, especially the world of the school. We have also seen how the context of adult–child interaction is a discourse situation that has its own unique characteristics and that, particularly in the early years, these characteristics serve to facilitate the child's participation in discourse, and provide information about other levels of language.

Discourse analysis can be a tool in helping to describe the difficulties displayed by pragmatically impaired children, and it can be shown how conversations between such children and their conversational partners can break down in various ways. Care must be taken in defining instances of inappropriacy, however. Because of the essentially 'fluid' nature of conversational discourse, and the impossibility of knowing every detail of the context and participants, it may be difficult to reach a satisfactory level of agreement as to what constitutes inappropriate conversational behaviour.

Note

We are grateful to Jennifer Reid for devising the question and responses used in exercise 3.4.

Chapter 4: Referring expressions

Key words: language in context, deixis, reference, deictic centre, time and space concepts, common ground, anaphora, ellipsis.

Aims

There are expressions in language, such as pronouns, which gain their specific meanings with reference to specific contexts. In a way, such expressions are relatively 'empty' semantically when they are out of context. To give an example, what does the word 'she' mean? From a semantic point of view it means 'a female animate being' (leaving aside, for the moment, the use of 'she' in reference to ships, cars and so on). In these terms, the expression 'she' can refer to any such 'being' in the world, but it clearly does not do so when used in a specific linguistic expression such as 'she is beautiful' (uttered when looking at a picture of a baby). In order to comprehend what the utterance means, it is necessary to realize that 'she' refers to the particular baby. Through this realization it is then possible for another person to take the conversation further ('Yes, she looks just like my Sharon as a baby'). The idea of specific linguistic expressions referring to context to gain their meaning is explored in this chapter.

Key questions:
What is deixis (deictic use of language)?
How does deictic use of language relate to people, time, space and social situations?
What does a deictic centre mean?
How does anaphoric and non-anaphoric usage differ?
How does indexicality develop?
Do language impaired children have difficulty with referring expressions?

68

How does indexicality relate to pragmatic impairment?
What is the clinical significance of referring expressions?

In a way, all expressions gain their meaning in context. At one level, the word 'cat' has a different meaning depending on which cat in the real world it refers to (for example, a pet or a tiger) or who uses the word (one who likes cats or one who does not). Yet, at another level, a more 'core' level, the word 'cat' refers to a particular subset of animals with particular identifying features, and only to these particular animals. In this latter sense, the meaning of the word 'cat' can be said to be relatively fixed. When we compare the word 'cat' to the word 'she', as discussed above, we can see that the meaning of the pronoun is more fluid. We already alluded to the fact that 'she' can refer not only to 'animate female beings', but also to inanimate objects such as 'ships' or 'cars', albeit more uncommonly. One might even choose to refer to one's computer as 'she'. So, what does 'she' mean semantically (that is, out of context)? It simply means 'a person or thing other than the speaker or the listener'. On hearing this pronoun, the listener would need to seek for a suitable referent which is other than the speaker or the listener. This search base is potentially very large. However, in communication, speakers normally try to produce their utterances in such a way that it is possible for the listener to locate referents for expressions without too much difficulty (see Chapters 6 and 7 further).

Background concepts and issues

Lund and Duchan (1993) look at reference from the point of view of how the listener is likely to have access to the referent. They talk about seven types of referring expressions. It is useful to start with these categories, since they come into play throughout this chapter.

1.   There are expressions for which the referent is to be found in the situational (physical/visual) context ('it's her, not her', accompanied by nods in appropriate directions). Following Halliday and Hasan (1976), these are called *exophoric expressions*.
2.   When using expressions such as 'I saw a cat in my garden', the phrase 'a cat' introduces a new referent into the listener's mind.
3.   When a referent has already been introduced in discourse and is then referred to again, the listener already has a representation of the referent and simply needs to access this in order to interpret the expression. So, if the above expression about the cat was followed by 'it dug up my flowers', the referent for 'it' would be accessed this way. Following Halliday and Hasan (1976) these are called *anaphoric*

expressions, which means that the referent is found in what has been previously mentioned.

4. There may be a situation where the referent is provided later on in discourse and hence the listener will need to keep it in mind until it can be resolved. An example of this would be: 'it's digging up my flowers again. That naughty cat', where the word 'it' in the first utterance refers to the cat in the second utterance. Using Halliday and Hasan's (1976) terminology, these are called *cataphoric expressions*, which means that the referent is found in a forthcoming utterance.

5. When we interpret the following short text, we need to use our world knowledge about court proceedings to assign referents to the phrases 'the judge' and 'the room'. In doing this, we engage in the cognitive process of inferencing and hence these types of expressions are called by Lund and Duchan *referring expressions requiring inferencing*. Text: 'The judge was ready to speak. Silence filled the room.'

6. In some situations, the listener may have more than one plausible interpretation for a referring expression and hence will need to disambiguate the referent. An example of this would be the following: 'A woman and a girl walked towards the school. Suddenly, *she* turned around'. These kinds of expression are called *referring expressions requiring disambiguation* by Lund and Duchan.

7. In the above example (6), it could be that in some situations the listener does not have enough information to find the referent for 'she', and hence cannot interpret it. Lund and Duchan call these *referring expressions that are uninterpretable*. While the referring expressions that require disambiguation become disambiguated, the uninterpretable referring expressions remain ambiguous.

The phenomena of referring expressions are interesting in the context of pragmatic language impairments. Being able to produce and comprehend such contextually determined meanings requires complex cognitive (including inferencing, metacognitive and theory of mind abilities), linguistic and social skills. The very nature of reference predicts problems for children who have difficulty using context in language processing. Literature on children's pragmatic impairments has suggested that one defining feature of such impairments may be difficulty in integrating linguistic and contextual information in an appropriate way, given the demands of the communicative situation (for example, McTear, 1985a; Bishop and Adams, 1991; Leinonen and Kerbel, 1999). The aim of this chapter is to give a brief overview of the phenomenon of referring expressions from the point of view of pragmatics and then explore the relevance of this for the understanding of the nature of pragmatic impairment in children.

Deixis

Deixis is a Greek word which means 'pointing' or 'indicating'. There are a finite number of words in English which gain their meaning by 'pointing to context'. All the personal pronouns can be used deictically (but see also non-deictic use, below). Similarly, the demonstrative pronouns 'this' or 'that' are deictic, as are words such as 'here' and 'there' and time references such as 'now', 'today' or 'tomorrow'. Furthermore, some verbs have a pointing function. The change of verb in the expression 'Are you *coming/going* over?' shows how the meanings of the verbs are anchored on the location of the speaker. Use of the verb 'come' indicates that the speaker is in the location that the listener is invited to, whereas the use of 'go' places the speaker somewhere else. Comparative forms such as 'I want something *different*' or 'Isn't there anything *warmer*?' also assume a point of reference (point of comparison) for their interpretation. The definite article 'the' has a deictic function in the sense that it tells the listener that what is being talked about is identifiable in context (for example, previously mentioned or commonly known). We will discuss deictic usage in detail, after first considering some general features of deixis.

One defining feature of all deictic expressions is that their reference is determined in relation to the *deictic centre* of the utterance. All deictic utterances have a deictic centre (also known as point of origin or 'origo') which helps to determine what the expression refers to. Let us explore this in the following exercise.

EXERCISE 4.1

In the following sentences, state what the italic (deictic) words refer to.

(a) I would like to buy *this*.
(b) I would like to buy *that*.
(c) Please put the present *here*.
(d) Please put the present *there*.
(e) I would like you to leave *now*.
(f) I would like you to leave *today*.
(g) I would like you to leave *tomorrow*.

Comment 4.1

(a) 'This' refers to 'something that is close to the speaker'.
(b) 'That' refers to 'something that is away from the speaker'.
(c) 'Here' refers to 'a place that is close to the speaker'.

(d) 'There' refers to 'a place that is away from the speaker'.
(e) 'Now' refers to 'at the time when the utterance is uttered'.
(f) 'Today' refers to 'the same day when the utterance is uttered'.
(g) 'Tomorrow' refers to 'the day after when the utterance is uttered'.

What the utterances (a) to (d) have in common is that they are 'anchored' to the place of the speaker. What this means is that when we hear 'this' or 'that' (or 'here' or 'there'), as in the above utterances, we know that the referent we need to identify is either close to or away from the speaker. We know where to look for the referent, and hence our search for the referent, and consequently the meaning of the expression, is constrained relative to the place of the speaker. If I was holding a melon in my hand and said to the greengrocer 'I would like to buy this', s/he would most likely not reach for another melon (or a cucumber or a turnip) on a shelf behind him/her but would correctly look for the referent near me and identify 'this' as referring to the melon in my hand rather than the purse in my other hand.

*　*　*　*　*　*

Types of deixis

The centre of a deictic utterance refers to the point at which the expression is 'anchored'. In the examples (a) to (d) above, the expressions are anchored in the place relative to the speaker. Levinson (1983) refers to this kind of deixis as *place deixis*. There are also some less obvious examples of place deixis – words such as come/go, bring/take, up/down and behind/in front of. These also hinge on the place of the speaker for their correct use and interpretation.

We can now see that the deictic centre (or 'anchorage') for the expressions in the utterances (e) to (g) is the time at which the utterances are uttered. Levinson (1983) refers to these kinds of expressions as *time deixis*. Time expressions are abstract relational concepts that require the ability to compare some point in time with the time of the utterance. Time expressions gain their meaning through this comparison. As such, time concepts are fluid or indeterminate rather than fixed or determinate. In some ways, time deixis is more indeterminate than place deixis in that it is not anchored to a physical situation, as place deixis is, but to an abstract concept of time. Hence, anyone who has difficulty with abstract concepts, and relationality, would most likely experience difficulty producing and comprehending time concepts.

There is a third type of deixis, which we have already had examples of but which was not illustrated in Exercise 4.1. Levinson (1983) calls this type *person deixis*. Person deixis includes personal pronouns and their various grammatical forms (for example, I, my, mine). The deictic centre for person deixis is the 'speaker'. For instance, 'I' means the speaker and 'you' the addressee and 's/he' neither the speaker nor the addressee (a third person). In this way, the referents for person deixis are found in relation to the person who uttered the expression.

Levinson (1983) discusses two further types of deixis which he terms *social deixis* and *discourse deixis*. Social deixis refers to the encoding of social distinctions relative to participant roles. An example of this would be the use of the second person pronoun in some languages (not English). In French and Finnish, for instance, there is a choice of two forms for the pronoun 'you' (French 'tu' or 'vous'; Finnish 'sinä' or 'te'). The choice is made on the basis of the speaker's social standing in relation to the addressee or the degree of familiarity between the speaker and the addressee. So, you would choose 'vous' or 'te' if you spoke to a person you did not know very well and 'tu' or 'sinä' if you were reasonably familiar with the speaker. In this way, the deictic centre for these pronouns is the social standing of the speaker relative to the addressee.

Discourse deixis refers to the use of expressions in reference to portions of the unfolding discourse. Examples of this would be expressions such as 'the *next* chapter' or '*this* paragraph is about ...'. In both of these examples, the deictic centre is the discourse location of the current utterance (that is, the current chapter, the current paragraph). Discourse conjunctions such as 'however', 'on the other hand' or 'furthermore' can also be considered deictic in character. What they indicate to the addressee is that what is to follow is to be interpreted as being in a particular meaning relationship to what has already been expressed. The relational nature of deixis is, again, very clear here.

Levinson (1983) raises an interesting general point about deixis. As speakers change, the deictic centres change too. They are, in fact, rather abruptly moved from speaker to speaker as conversation progresses. As the whole of the deictic system hinges on the speaker (for all the types of deixis, except discourse deixis), it is in a state of flux in conversations (as a consequence of speaker changes). Certain flexibility of thought (cognition) is needed in order for one to be able to follow such switches of deictic centres and for one to be able to adjust one's own production and interpretation of utterances accordingly. One could imagine this being problematic for children with certain types of cognitive deficit.

Gestural and symbolic deixis

Deixis can pick out its referent *gesturally* or *symbolically*. In the former case, the referent can be established only when there is a physical (visual, auditory or tactile) monitoring of the situation in which the expression occurs. In the following expressions, the deictic usage is gestural: 'Put it

here', 'Don't touch *it'*. '*He* is *his* boss' (speaker nods in appropriate directions). Symbolic usage of deixis, on the other hand, requires for its interpretation only general or basic knowledge of the location and time of the
utterance (and sometimes some social knowledge). When you receive a
postcard from a friend and it says 'It's beautiful *here'*, you need to know
only that the person is away from their usual place of habitation and that
'here' refers to that place. You may, of course, know that it is a particular
place, say Devon or a particular town in Devon, or even a particular
clifftop on the Devon coast which you have both visited previously, but in
all these cases, if the card does not state what 'here' refers to (see
anaphora below), the use of the word 'here' is symbolic. One could
suppose that gestural and symbolic use of deixis encompass different
degrees of abstraction, gestural being less abstract than symbolic, and
hence, differential cognitive demands may be placed on a person when
they are processed.

Non-deictic usage and anaphora

One further important point to recognize is that not all occurrences of
words that can be used deictically are always deictic (that is, are not
'pointing to context for interpretation'). In the expression '*You* never
know what will happen next', 'you' can gain its meaning either through
reference to a particular person (that is, you specifically rather than other
people) or to the general body of people (that is, one never knows). In
the former case, 'you' is used deictically and in the latter it is being used
non-deictically.

EXERCISE 4.2

In this exercise your task is to decide whether the italicized words are
used deictically or non-deictically and, if they are used deictically, it is your
task to say what type of deixis is involved.

   (a) *You* and *you*, out.
   (b) *There* is some doubt about *that*.
   (c) *Now* never lasts for long enough.
   (d) I went to *this* great party.

Comment 4.2

   (a) Both words are deictic; instances of person and gestural deixis.
   (b) 'There' is non-deictic; 'that' is an instance of discourse deixis if

we consider 'that' as referring to the content of a previous
expression.
(c) 'Now' is non-deictic; it does not refer to any particular point in
time.
(d) 'This' is non-deictic; it is used instead of the indefinite article 'a'.

* * * * * *

A further way of using pronouns (personal and demonstrative) non-deictically is that of anaphoric reference (or anaphora). In this kind of reference, the pronoun points to a prior expression in the discourse for
interpretation. The pronoun picks out the same referent as the person or
thing previously mentioned. In the example, 'Mary liked fast cars. So, *she*
bought a sports car', the word 'she' gains its specific meaning by reference
to the previously mentioned word 'Mary'. In processing terms, the difference between deixis and anaphora is that for deixis the search space for
the referent is potentially more indeterminate (or less constrained)
whereas in the case of anaphora the referent has been already explicitly
stated, so potentially the referent is more easily available.

Ellipsis

Similar to anaphoric reference is ellipsis in language. Halliday and Hasan
(1976) discuss both of these within the notion of cohesion. It is not
customary to discuss ellipsis in a chapter on deixis or referring expressions, but we decided to include a short discussion of it here for the
reason that elliptical utterances, like anaphoric reference, gain their
meaning through reference to other expressions. In this way, processes
underlying production and comprehension of elliptical utterances are
likely to be similar to anaphora and deixis. Elliptical utterances are
grammatically and conceptually incomplete, and hence one needs to
search outside the utterance for the 'complete' interpretation. In the
following example, the italicized utterances are elliptical:

A: I had chicken for dinner.
B: *What else?*
A: *Chips and peas.*

The italicized utterances clearly cannot be interpreted without reference to the previous utterance 'I had chicken for dinner'. One needs to
expand the elliptical utterances to something like 'What else, in addition to
chicken, did you have for dinner?' and 'I had chips and peas with the
chicken for my dinner'. Language users are clearly able to engage in such
'conceptual expansions' when interpreting elliptical utterances. We will
discuss in Chapter 7 how we may go about explaining elliptical utterances.

Thinking about other people's minds

What all referring expressions have in common from the speaker's point of view is that s/he needs to be able to judge whether the addressee is able to recover the intended referent. In the case of gestural deixis, it is necessary to ensure that the addressee has access (visual, auditory or tactile) to the physical world being referred to. When symbolic deixis is used, an assessment needs to be made of the addressee's knowledge of the world and how accessible this is in the given context. In a way, the speaker needs to assess what knowledge the addressee is able to access and whether this is sufficient for recovering the intended referent. It is not uncommon, particularly in close relationships, for one to assume unreasonably that the other person is almost able to know one's thoughts and hence referring expressions which cannot be (easily) interpreted are produced. The ability to make judgements about others' knowledge and minds connects with 'theory of mind' abilities, and hence people with such social cognitive difficulties may well have difficulty with referring expressions.

Why does language have deixis (or referring expressions in general)? There would be less chance for miscommunication if we spelled out in full what we mean. In this way, the addressee would not need to search for referents and other information in the context in order to work out the intended meaning. They would simply have to decode what is being said. Language use could have evolved to be completely explicit, and consequently long-winded and repetitive, but it did not. Why not? The human brain has evolved the capacity to process implicit information in an efficient way and hence the input does not need to be explicit. If it were, it would be completely unnecessarily so. Communication via implicit means, one aspect of which involves deictic use of language, is something the human brain is customized for and in normal circumstances able to do highly efficiently.

Exercise 4.3

Here are some statements and hypotheses about referring expressions and possible difficulty that one might have with them. Your task is to say whether these are potentially valid/true or invalid/false, and why.

(a) Deictic centre changes in conversations.
(b) Children who have difficulty with relationality could have difficulty with deixis.
(c) Pronouns are always deictic.
(d) Theory of mind difficulties could be reflected in difficulty with referring expressions.

(e) The search base for referents for deixis is potentially larger than the search base for anaphora.

(f) Difficulty in using context in production and comprehension of meaning could be reflected in difficulty with referring expressions.

Comment 4.3

(a) It is *true* that the point at which deictic utterances are anchored (the deictic centre) changes as speakers change. This is a simple consequence of the fact that the speaker is the point of anchorage for all types of deixis (except discourse deixis) and hence speaker change effects change of the deictic centre.

(b) This is a *valid* hypothesis. Deixis is a relational concept in the sense that in order to find the intended referent one needs to assess how the referent is placed in relation to the deictic centre. For instance, to find the referent for 'that' in the utterance 'How much is that?' one needs to realize that the referent is away from the speaker. As we also mentioned above, some of the relationships involved are more abstract (for example, time deixis) than others (for example, place deixis).

(c) This is *false* since pronouns can be used deictically or non-deictically. In the latter, there is no pointing to situational context for interpretation. Anaphoric use of pronouns is non-deictic in the sense that the referent is found in what has been previously said.

(d) This is a *valid* hypothesis. To produce and comprehend deictic utterances one needs to make an assessment about the other person's ability to recover the intended referent.

(e) This is *true* in that anaphoric referents have a verbally given referent whereas the referents for deixis have to be found in physical or mental contexts and hence deixis is potentially less constrained. However, it is true that in cooperative interactions the speaker aims to produce utterances in such a manner as to facilitate the identification of referents by the addressee (see Chapters 6 and 7 further).

(f) This hypothesis is *valid* in that referring expressions are completely dependent on context for their meaning.

* * * * * *

As we have seen, referring expressions, such as deixis, anaphora and ellipsis, gain their meaning in context. Hence, the ability to take into account many different aspects of the context in which utterances occur is essential in appropriate production and comprehension of referring expressions. From what we know about pragmatic language difficulties and what pragmatic theory would predict, referring expressions may well be problematic for those children who have pragmatic impairments. Before looking at what the literature suggests of such children, let us first see how the ability to handle referring expressions develops.

Developmental notes

Children's earliest pointing behaviours (with or without vocalizations), well before the age of one, are interpreted as having communicative import (proto-conversations, Bateson, 1975). These expressions identify some entity in the child's environment and tend to serve the function of directing others' attention to this entity. In this way, they can be said not to have a truly referential function (Atkinson, 1979). Some researchers have referred to them as 'proto-declaratives' (Bates, 1979) (see also Chapter 2). Specific deictic words (namely 'this' and 'that') tend to be among children's first words, but they do not have a speaker perspective attached to them and hence they are not truly deictic in nature. As we noted above, deictic expressions are anchored on the speaker and gain some of their meaning through this anchorage. As children start to use deictic expressions, they use them first non-deictically, simply to refer to items in their environment without apparent regard for the speaker as a deictic centre. This is evident in the following example from a child (bilingual Finnish/English) of 3;1. The child is inside the house and is pointing through the window into the garden.

Minun näki äsken kissan *tällä* ulkona. (should be *tuolla* ulkona)
I just saw a cat *here* outside. (should be *there* outside)

In this example the child uses the wrong place deictic term, which reflects either lack of understanding of the speaker as the deictic centre in the use of these words or difficulty in determining what could be counted as being close or far. As Lund and Duchan (1993) point out, distance being relative, the boundary between close or far may be difficult for children to gauge in some situations when they first start making such judgements.

As the speaker is the anchorage to all deictic usage, it is not surprising that person deixis develops first. Clark (1978) noted that 2 year olds were already developing the contrast between 'I' and 'you'. She observed two stages in this development before appropriate usage. First of all, children tended to use 'I' without a contrast to 'you'. At this 'stage' the child need not be aware of the deictic principle that pronoun use reflects who is speaking and who is listening. Then, some children were observed to use both 'I' and 'you', but reversing the usage. In other words, children at this stage would use 'you' referring to themselves and 'I' referring to others.

This would reflect a principle whereby a child would equate pronoun usage with name usage (that is, I = mummy; you = the child, as this is how they would hear the pronouns used to them). Again the speaker principle is not observed here. Such reversals are thought to be very rare and, in fact, Chiat (1986) believes that normally developing children do not equate pronouns with names, but are capable from a young age of shifting reference according to speaker change. The fine-tuning of person deixis acquisition to include appropriate use of gender marking (he/she) continues to develop through the early school years.

Less is known about the development of deictic systems other than person deixis. The deictic terms associated with proximity to speaker (place deixis, here/there, this/that) tend to start developing after 'person deixis' even though they are used non-deictically from an early age (see above). The deictic prepositions 'in front of' and 'behind' tend to emerge before other place deixis. As Lund and Duchan (1993) observe, these prepositions tend to be easier to acquire than the other place deixis and this may be aided by the prepositions having non-deictic usage too. Some objects have an intrinsic 'front' and 'back' (for example, television, house, bike) and reference to the front/back of these objects is non-deictic, since one does not need to figure out where the speaker or addressee is positioned ('Look in front of the television'). Children comprehend the non-deictic usage of these terms relatively early. However, the 'front' of a tree changes as a function of where the speaker and the addressee are positioned. Hence, the front becomes the back as one moves around. This usage is deictic and is acquired later than the non-deictic usage. There is also a tendency for the 'close' terms (here/this) to be acquired before the 'far' terms (there/that). In more general terms, the acquisition of place deixis suggests that the learning process is aided by 'fixedness of meaning' from which the more fluid aspects of meaning arise.

It takes the longest for children to acquire time deixis. Children as old as 8 have been observed to get their yesterdays and tomorrows wrong. Time is the least tangible and fixed of all the deictic meanings. As Piaget (1926) observed, the concept of time, as well as causality, is acquired relatively late in cognitive development. Piaget has further suggested that children understand sequencing of time before they understand duration, which is reflected in their earlier understanding of words such as 'before' and 'after' as compared with words such as 'until' or 'since'. Children start to use the past tense forms of verbs after 3 years of age and in this way indicate the beginnings of the coding of time in language. The use of the words 'now' and 'tomorrow' has been observed from 3 years onwards, too. However, 'tomorrow' tends to simply mean 'not now, but in the future'. Interestingly, even though children use past tense verb endings to describe past events, the concept of 'yesterday' is difficult to grasp. In

Piaget's terms, this again would reflect the distinction of time as a sequential concept and one that encompasses duration.

Referential usage in discourse (anaphora, cataphora and ellipsis) is another area that children acquire over time. In her study of 2–5-year-old children's narratives, Bennett-Kastor (1983) found that children as young as 2 were able to reiterate a noun phrase in order to provide referential linkage. With age, children moved from the repetition of noun phrases to providing a pronoun for the already mentioned referent. However, in a longitudinal study of 10 children between 2;0 and 3;6, Peterson and Dodsworth (1991) noted that although children's noun specification improved with age, when introducing new nouns, about one in five was still ambiguous at age 3;6. Flavell (1985) has similarly observed young children's tendency to use ambiguous pronouns and nouns when speaking. Young children frequently underspecify, especially when excited or upset (for example, the child who comes in from the playground and says 'he hit me'). Peterson and Dodsworth further found that comparative reference and ellipsis emerged later than the other reference categories identified in Halliday and Hasan's (1976) framework, even though these were also already present by age 3. The most common way of signalling referential linkage was by lexical means, which has been shown to decline with age. School-aged children have been shown to use a greater variety of linking than the young subjects of Peterson and Dodsworth. A further interesting observation in this study was that the children's use of ellipsis declined with age, and this was shown to be a function of the children becoming individual narrators as opposed to joint narrators with an adult, when they respond to adult's prompting by an elliptical utterance.

When comprehending utterances, Umstead and Leonard (1983) observed that even 3-year-olds were able to locate antecedents for pronouns in short stories and that this ability improved with age (3–5-year-olds). They further found that when the anaphora-antecedent pairs were in the same sentence, children's accuracy improved as compared with their accuracy across sentence pairs. This may reflect a difference between grammatical and pragmatic processing of anaphora. Children's ability to handle anaphora in narratives is discussed further in Chapter 5.

Referential communication tasks have been used to examine children's ability to communicate to others distinguishing features of referents. In these tasks a child has to describe to another person items in such a way that the other person can pick them out from an array of possible items, which have shared attributes (for example, colour, shape, 'the blue, round one'). The important point is to pay attention to the critical dimensions that distinguish the particular item from other items in the array. Earlier interpretations (Glucksberg and Krauss, 1967) of this paradigm suggest that the task sheds light on children's understanding of what the other person needs to know in order to pick out the intended item. Later work (Bishop and Adams, 1991; Leinonen and Letts, 1997a) has shown that the task reflects how children are engaged in a complex cognitive analysis of feature salience and integration of information in order to identify a particular referent uniquely. Lloyd (1990) gives a short historical account of research with normal child populations using this paradigm.

Clinical populations

It has been recognized for some time that children with language, and particularly pragmatic, difficulties may have difficulty with the use of referring expressions. Prutting and Kirchner (1987) examined the extent to which language-disordered children were judged to have difficulty with each of the 30 parameters of the *Pragmatic Protocol* (Prutting and Kirchner, 1983). They found that 'specificity/accuracy' and 'cohesion' were most frequently marked inappropriate in conversations involving language-disordered children (71% and 55% of the subjects having difficulty in these categories). 'Specificity/accuracy' refers to overuse of unestablished referents and lexical items that hinder understanding, and 'cohesion' includes reference as one of its categories. Other researchers have commented on similar difficulties with insufficient specificity (for example, Damico, 1985; Jones, Smedley and Jennings, 1986). Bishop and Adams (1989) noted that language impaired children with pragmatic difficulties had problems with producing the right amount of information in order for the listener to understand the expression appropriately. In part, this difficulty was related to referential usage, where the referent was not easy to recover.

A study by Bishop and Adams (1991), using a referential communication paradigm, found that SLI children were poorer than age-matched controls at giving relevant information. They more frequently failed to give information about the critical dimension (for example, a curly or straight tail of a white or black dog/cat) which would have enabled the investigator to identify the correct picture. This was not considered a reflection of the children's expressive abilities. A subgroup of the language-disordered children who matched the profile of 'semantic-pragmatic disorder' did not perform any more poorly than the other language-disordered children. This was considered somewhat surprising since these same children had difficulty providing the right amount of information in open-ended conversational settings. It is suggested that the cognitive and social demands of a conversational situation outweigh the complexity of the referential communication task. In line with this, Leinonen and Letts (1997a) observed that seven children (age range

6;4–8;9) who were considered to have pragmatic difficulties were able to give and receive instructions in a task that required them to describe a picture so that the other person was able to manipulate a set of objects (critical dimensions: colour, size, number – for example, 'put a large, blue brick in the box'). What the children found problematic, however, was when the experimenter gave an inadequate instruction (for example, 'put the pencil in a cup', where the colour of the pencil is left unspecified). Although the age-matched control children (age range 6;3–7;9) asked for clarification, the pragmatically impaired children did not do so even after they were given feedback about the inadequate instruction. This suggests that looking out for critical dimensions of referents in more communicative situations may be problematic for children with pragmatic impairments. It was also observed in this study that only the pragmatically impaired children specified unnecessary dimensions when giving instructions to the adult. For instance, some of them specified the colour of the plate when this was unnecessary as there was only one plate. This, again, shows some insensitivity to the notion of a critical dimension.

A referential communication study of 10 children with SLI and 10 children with normal language development by Johnston, Smith and Box (1997) made the important observation that the cognitive load associated with certain aspects of the task influenced how the children communicated the needed information to the listener. Whereas both groups were equally successful in the task, the description of size (as opposed to colour) proved difficult for the groups. It is argued that size is a relational concept and as such a cognitively more demanding concept to manipulate than colour (see also the discussion on relationality and time in this chapter). The study makes the further point that the complexity of communication tasks which children engage in influences children's use of the language forms that they know, and hence failure in linguistic performance may reflect cognitive (momentary) overload.

In their study of 8 SLI, 10 autistic and 8 normally functioning children, matched on language age (including mean length of utterance (MLU), receptive vocabulary and syntax), Baltaxe and D'Angiola (1996) examined the correct and incorrect use of reference (personal pronouns, demonstrative pronouns and comparatives). The children were studied in a dialogue situation. The normal children produced many more correct uses than the clinical populations. It is suggested that the problem of referencing in the clinical groups may be indicative of deviance rather than delay. Interestingly, however, the autistic children differed from the SLI group in that they produced many more incorrect uses, and these uses were also qualitatively different. Although the SLI and normal groups produced mainly omission errors, errors of non-identification and selection were common in the autistic group. Baltaxe and D'Angiola hypothesize that errors where a pronoun is present but cannot be identified (non-identification error), or errors where a child has selected an incorrect pronoun (selection error), are more detrimental for the listener than omission errors. They further suggest that omission and selection errors may be developmentally interpreted as reflecting the emergence of context-sensitive grammatical rules, whereas non-identification errors are related to the development of social and pragmatic skills. This is then interpreted to mean that the reference errors made by the autistic children may have a non-linguistic basis, whereas the errors of the normal and SLI children are likely to be linguistically based. Baltaxe and D'Angiola further noted that 'pronoun reversal' (that is, the use of I/me for you), which was once considered a stable characteristic of autism, was not a notable feature of the data (see also Jordan, 1989).

Working within the relevance theory framework of Sperber and Wilson (1995), Leinonen and Kerbel (1999) found that it was possible to locate difficulties in reference assignment in the language of three children with pragmatic difficulties. However, referencing seemed to be less of a problem than other aspects of pragmatic functioning (see Chapter 7 further). The children found those aspects of pragmatic meaning more difficult than reference assignment which involved complex contextual processing whereby information needed to be brought together from a number of sources in order to arrive at a relevant interpretation. Elliptical utterances provide a good example of utterances that are subject to such complex processing. Many examples can be found in the literature which indicate a similar kind of difficulty with elliptical utterances by children with pragmatic problems (for example, Bishop and Adams, 1989; Mills, Pulles and Witten, 1992; Leinonen, 1995). The production and interpretation of referring expressions can be seen to be intrinsically linked with one's ability to activate context in a relevant way in language processing (see Chapter 7).

In a study of cohesion of the narratives of 20 normal and 20 language-disordered children (aged 7;6–10;6), Liles (1985) found that language-disordered children used significantly fewer personal pronoun ties than the normal controls. Instead they used many more demonstrative reference ties and lexical ties. Liles suggests that it may be that 'chaining' of personal referents across a narrative causes difficulty for the disordered group and that this difficulty may partly reflect these subjects' late acquisition of pronominal use. The use of the developmentally early demonstrative pronouns and the developmentally early strategy of signalling connectedness by lexical choice supports Liles' explanation. However, the language-disordered group performed similarly to the normal controls in their use of referents (and cohesive ties in general) when they told the narrative to an uninformed listener (one who had not seen the film that formed the basis of the narrative) rather than an informed listener. This showed that despite their difficulties with pronominal reference, the language-disordered children were able to adjust their language output for the needs of the listener. Hence, their social and pragmatic functioning would not be said to be impaired.

Oakhill and Yuill (1986) found in their study of 24 skilled and less-skilled comprehenders (mean age 7;9 in both groups) that the less-skilled group found it difficult to answer questions about pronoun antecedents. The subjects were, for instance, to fill in the missing pronouns in short scenarios such as 'Sally gave her shoes to Ben as a present because ... needed them' (p.32). The input was controlled for gender cues and differed in terms of inferential complexity. It was found that gender cues did not help the less-skilled comprehenders. Interestingly, the comprehension was also not helped by allowing the children to refer back to the given scenarios. Hence, memory limitations did not seem to account for the results. The increasing inferential complexity of the task widened the differences between the two groups further, suggesting that, at least in part, the difficulties of the less-skilled comprehenders could be attributed to processing of complex information (see Chapter 6 further).

Clinical data

There follows an extract from a conversation between an adult (one of the authors) and Simon, a 13-year-old boy with pragmatic difficulties (also discussed in Chapters 5 and 6). These data come from Smith and Leinonen (1992:266–7) (see also Leinonen and Kerbel, 1999).

EXERCISE 4.4

Your task is to discuss the referential usage by both Simon and the adult in relation to the italicized pronouns. There are other referring expressions in this extract too, but as we will see, the pronouns alone will give us a fair amount to discuss. We have also excluded the personal pronouns 'I' and 'you', as these are not problematic for Simon. Your task is to comment on what the pronouns mean and whether Simon's responses show understanding of the intended meanings. Before the conversation took place, Simon had written a story for the adult, which the adult had just read (A= adult; C = child).

    A: That's a good story, but I find *it* (1) quite difficult to understand. Why do
        you think I find *it* (1) difficult to understand ?
    C: I don't know.
    A: Is *it* (2) because I have never seen *it* (3)?

C: No.

A: No. Do you think I should understand *it* (4) from *this* (5) ?

C: Yes.

A: Umm 'cos I am not always sure what 'they' ... 'cos you say *they* (6) did something and *they* (7) did something. I am not always sure what '*they*' (8) refers to. 'Cos I don't know.

C: Yes.

A: I haven't seen the film. Do you understand what I am saying?

C: Yes.

A: So how do you think you could make *it* (9) sometimes more understandable?

C: Don't know.

A: Maybe instead of saying *they* (10) did something and *they* (11) did such and such you could say who *they* (12) are.

C: The people?

A: Is *it* (13) all about the people?

C: Yes.

A: The people did ... Is *it* (14) a group of people?

C: Yes.

A: Um er OK. How about the end? Is *that* (15) 'soldiers'? (points to the word 'soldiers' in the story)

C: Guarding.

A: Guarding. So *he* (16) cut the rope? (points to the word 'he' in the story)

C: Yes.

A: Who is *he* (17)?

C: Indiana Jones.

A: Oh Indiana Jones. Well, you didn't say did ya?

C: (laughing) What?

A: You didn't say Indiana Jones, did you?

C: At the start of *it* (18)?

A: Where?

C: You mean should've *it* (19) been mentioned?

A: Yeah. Don't you think?

C: Think *it* (20) should be all mentioned all in the story as well?

A: Well *it* (21) should have been said in the beginning 'cos I didn't know *this* (22) was about Indiana Jones, 'cos I haven't seen the film, have I?

C: No

A: 'cos otherwise I didn't know who *he* (23) was

Comment 4.4

The communicative problem that the adult and Simon attempt to solve in this example arises because Simon uses pronouns in his written text without giving the listener access to the appropriate antecedents. It is interesting to note the various strategies and rephrasing that the adult attempts in order to get Simon to see what the problem is with his story, and indeed Simon shows some realization of the difficulty towards the end of the extract. Given that the adult is aware that antecedents for pronouns are problematic for Simon, the adult nevertheless uses pronouns herself in almost every utterance. This is not likely to facilitate Simon's comprehension. Let us look at the referential usage in this example in some detail.

- *it* (1) – These two 'its' refer to the story written by Simon. It is not clear from Simon's reply whether or not he has comprehended these.
- *it* (2) and *it* (3) – The first of these means something like 'my difficulty with the understanding of your story' and the second means 'the film that I as the reader assume you are writing about'. These are very complicated references, and both are in the same sentence. Simon does not show comprehension of the intended meanings here. This is likely to reflect, at least partly, difficulty with assigning referents for the two pronouns.
- *it* (4) and *this* (5) – The 'it' refers again to Simon's story and the word 'this' refers to the actual written imprint of the story (that is, deictic meaning). It is difficult to infer from Simon's minimal response whether he has or has not understood the meanings of the pronouns.
- *they* (6), (7) and (8) – These three pronouns mean something like the word 'they' as used in the story
- *it* (9) – This 'it' refers to the story again, but is potentially very confusing because the nearest possible antecedent is 'the film' in the adult's previous utterance. It is not possible to infer from Simon's utterance whether he has understood the referent.
- *they* (10), (11) and 12 – These three pronouns mean, like before, 'the word they as used in the story'. Simon shows now some understanding of the problem: that he needs to provide a referent for the word 'they', which he makes an attempt at doing. Unfortunately, his answer 'the people' is not helpful because it is not specific enough. The use of the definite article 'the' also shows lack of understanding by Simon that 'the' means that the other person should know 'the people' (that is, 'the' indicates shared knowledge).
- *it* (13) – This refers to the story. It is difficult to infer Simon's comprehension from the minimal answer.
- *it* (14) – This refers to the aforementioned 'people'. Interestingly, the adult is using this reference even though she does not know who the people are (that is, is faking understanding).
- *that* (15) – The adult is now pointing to the word 'soldiers' and the word 'that' refers to the actual word on the page (that is, is deictic). It does not seem from Simon's utterance that he has understood this reference, but rather Simon seems to be reacting to the word 'soldiers' by providing a suitably related word to it.
- *he* (16) and *he* (17) – The adult uses the first 'he' to refer to the word

'he' written in the story, and the second 'he' is used to refer to a person still unknown to the adult, but which is the same 'he' who Simon said cut the rope in the story.

- *it* (18) – The adult uses the word 'it' here to refer to the story.
- *it* (19) and (20) – Simon uses 'it' here to refer to Indiana Jones, which the adult understands. Curiously, Simon does not use the pronoun 'he'. Because of this, it may be that Simon is using 'it' in a more abstract sense to refer to the idea of 'people who are included in a story should be mentioned'.
- *it* (21) – The adult uses 'it' to mean 'referencing in general' rather than Indiana Jones.
- *this* (22) – The adult refers here to 'the story'.
- *he* (23) – The adult refers to Indiana Jones.

Linguistic interpretation

It is interesting to note the number of different uses just a few pronouns are put to in a short extract of conversation. It is difficult to say in hindsight whether the various usages of the pronouns by the adult had hindered Simon's comprehension, but if we accept that Simon has pragmatic difficulties, then comprehension of the shifting contextual meanings of the pronouns could be potentially problematic for him. We can see from the exercise that the pronouns in this conversation are used in a number of ways. There are several metalinguistic/metacommunicative meanings of them, for instance when 'it' is used to refer to Simon's story and when 'it' (2) refers to the adult's lack of understanding of his story. The three uses of 'they' (6,7, 8) are also metalinguistic in the sense that they refer to the word 'they' as used in the story. To work out the meanings of such pronouns requires complex metalinguistic and cognitive processing. In a similar way, to assign a referent for the second 'it' in the sentence 'Is it because I have not seen it?' requires Simon to realize that the antecedent for the word 'it' has not been mentioned but is in the mind of the adult in so far that the adult has hypothesized that Simon's story is about a film. This again is a complex process requiring the ability to work out what the other person has worked out in their own mind. Again, it would not be surprising if Simon had not been able to do this, given that pragmatically impaired children may have social cognitive deficits. There are also gestural deictic uses of 'this' and 'that' (5, 15) in the data, where the adult is drawing upon the written context when trying to get Simon to understand what she means.

The adult succeeds in getting Simon to tell her what the story is about by asking the question 'Who is he?'. It is interesting to explore why this sentence would succeed when the others had not. By pointing to the word 'he' in the actual written text when asking 'So he cut the rope?' the adult is making it easier for Simon to know which 'he' she has trouble with. It then seems easier to assign a referent to the rapidly following 'who is he?'. Simon then shows awareness of the importance of enabling the listener to assign referents to pronouns. By saying, 'At the start of it?', 'You mean should've it been mentioned?' and 'Think it should be all mentioned all in the story as well?', Simon indicates some understanding of the problem the reader of his story was experiencing and in this way he shows some metacommunicative awareness.

It is clear from the clinical data explored here that pronouns do indeed gain meaning in context and that there are different levels of complexity involved in reference assignment. It is also fairly apparent that children who have difficulty with contextual aspects of meaning and children with cognitive deficits would find complex resolution of referents problematic. These data have also demonstrated how thought could be usefully given to the kind of linguistic input that pragmatically impaired children receive and how this could hinder or facilitate their performance.

Clinical interpretation

Assessment issues

The adult's response to Simon's story, and the evident difficulty she has in understanding it, point to a problem that is common with many language impaired children, that of underspecification of referents. Simon uses pronouns for which the referent is not clear to the reader (or listener). Reasons for this problem may differ, however, from child to child. Many language impaired children have difficulties with vocabulary, either with acquiring new words quickly and accurately, or with reproducing (or retrieving) the words that they know. As a result, in order to maintain communication uninterrupted, they may replace unknown vocabulary items with pronouns, leaving the listener confused as to what exactly is being talked about. In order to investigate this possibility, standardized vocabulary tests may be used. Ideally, both a receptive vocabulary test, such as the British Picture Vocabulary Scales (Dunn et al., 1997), and an expressive vocabulary test such as the Renfrew Word Finding Picture Vocabulary Test (Renfrew, 1995) or the Test of Word Finding (German, 1986) would be administered. By comparing receptive and expressive performance, it can be ascertained whether difficulties lie more with acquiring and retaining vocabulary, or with retrieving words already acquired. If vocabulary proves to be a problem, then remediation aimed at fostering vocabulary growth (or word retrieval) would be an appropriate first step.

Another situation in which a language impaired individual may overuse pronouns, to the detriment of listener/reader comprehension, is if s/he is overloaded by the demands of the linguistic task. This could apply if grammar of some complexity is involved, or, perhaps in this case, if the medium is writing, which a child may find more demanding than speaking. Bypassing the need to specify referents clearly will cut the processing load, allowing the child to focus on the aspects that s/he finds difficult. A way of investigating this would be to compare the child's performance on tasks involving minimal processing load (such as an expressive vocabulary test where one-word naming responses are all that is required) with his/her performance when producing longer, more complex utterances. This exercise could also be applied to writing, where the child writes down single names for things and this is compared with more discursive writing.

However, children with difficulties of a more pragmatic nature may lack the necessary skills of how to use pronoun and other deictic forms adequately. They may not be sensitive to the listener's state of knowledge and how best to make themselves understood. From Simon's responses to the adult probes in this extract, it would certainly seem to be the case that he has difficulties in this area. If a child persistently has problems with referring expressions in the absence of any obvious influences that relate to vocabulary acquisition or processing load, then remediation focused directly on this area may well be helpful, provided that the vocabulary issue has been thoroughly addressed.

Therapy and management

Where a child (like Simon) shows evidence of difficulty in handling refer-ring expressions, the principles involved need to be made explicit and plenty of practice given. Simon shows that he is beginning to gain some insight (albeit limited) into his difficulty when he asks if Indiàna Jones' name should have been mentioned at various points. One problem with the extract given here is that the subject matter is complex. Considerable thought has to be given as to what exactly the various pronouns used might be referring to, and the adult finds it hard to avoid using potentially confusing referring expressions as well. Plainly, getting the child to describe an action-packed film that the adult has not seen may not be a good way to start. From an assessment point of view, however, this task does give a very vivid picture of Simon's problems.

Simple accounts, such as recounting a story about cartoon pictures or describing a more routine event that has happened in school, may be useful, with more complex events being used as the child gains in awareness. There is a need to challenge the child where referents are not clear, and to indicate how he or she can clarify the situation. Although it is useful if the listener knows something about the subject matter used in such exercises, it is important that communication is real, so that the child can see the impact of underspecification in real communicative situations. If he or she knows that the listener already knows a story, for example, the need for clear referring expressions no longer applies. It may be useful to have the child give an account to a third party (for example, another child or adult) while being prompted and helped by the therapist. Older children may write down a story for a third person to read. Letts and Reid (1994) give an account of a case study of a child who was given help with appropriate specification.

At the same time, any child who has difficulty using referring expressions is also likely to have difficulty understanding less obvious expressions as used by other people. The extract given above is full of examples of the adult using pronouns whose referents may be quite clear to more sophisticated language users, but which for Simon are likely to pose problems. A degree of monitoring by adults of their own referring expressions will be of benefit, and may continue to be needed even after the child begins to make some progress. There are places in the extract where the adult could have replaced *it* (for example, 9, 13) with 'your story', or (for example, 23) with 'people's names' or 'Indiana's name'. A rule of thumb might be to use pronouns only where the antecedent is the nearest possible one, as occurs in the adult's opening turn:

> that's a good story, but I find *it* (the story) quite difficult to understand. Why
> do you think I find *it* (the story) difficult to understand?

On the other hand, children will have to learn to handle comprehension of referring expressions, so perhaps one should at times use pronouns and referring expressions in the manner that they are used in 'real' communication, perhaps together with some explanation as to what they mean. Self-monitoring is, of course, difficult to maintain all the time, but modification where the child indicates that s/he has failed to understand should be possible. This also gives a good model; the child sees that the appropriate response to incomprehension is to modify one's utterance, and that a potentially helpful way of doing this is to specify the pronoun referents more clearly.

Summary

It is clear that expressions which gain their meaning through reference to context, either linguistic or non-linguistic, involve complex pragmatic processing of language. We have shown in this chapter that referring expressions can be said to encompass deictic expressions, ellipsis and anaphora. The concepts of time and space are central to deictic meaning, and through this we see a close connection with cognitive processing. Similarly, the need to build and maintain contexts in referent interpretation, for instance when expanding elliptical utterances, involves complex integration of information and memory skills. The development of referring ability starts early, pre-linguistically, and continues through the school years by continuing refinement of one's understanding of time deixis particularly. Children with language and other developmental disorders have been observed to both underspecify and overspecify referents, but those with particular pragmatic difficulties are likely to have a more substantial and sustained difficulty with referring expressions. This area requires further inquiry and research.

Chapter 5: Narratives and story telling

Key words: narrative production, story telling, coherence, referential usage, orientation, personal significance, macro and micro levels.

Aims

Telling a story is an activity in which children engage from a very early age and one which demonstrates children's increasing sophistication in handling context and knowledge for the purpose of communicating messages to other people. It requires a multitude of skills and competencies, and the study of children's narrative production and comprehension provides a good way of examining children's pragmatic functioning (see also Chapter 6). This chapter aims to explore the following:

Key questions:
What is a coherent narrative?
What kind of content is needed in a narrative?
What is the role of the topic and world knowledge in narrative production?
What skills are involved in story telling?
How does narrative skill develop?
What are language-disordered children like as narrators?
What are pragmatically impaired children like as narrators?
How does narrative ability relate to other pragmatic skills?
How do narratives fit into clinical management of communication disorders?

The value of studying narratives in the clinical context is highlighted by Liles (1993). Narratives tell us about:

• children's world experience and knowledge and how these are structured and represented

- children's cognitive skills that shape the content and structure of narratives
- the ability of children to take the communicative needs of others into account
- the skill with which children use linguistic form for communicative purposes.

A narrative requires children to operate both in the here and now and in the past, the future and imaginary worlds. It requires children to integrate information for specific purposes and to maintain integration and coherence over a period of time. Narrative, in even its most elementary form, is a relatively high-level cognitive, social and linguistic operation. It is therefore not too remarkable that the skill develops slowly through childhood into adolescence and adulthood and how those with various linguistic and non-linguistic impairments may have difficulty in producing coherent narratives.

Narratives have a central role in children's everyday lives, particularly in the school context. This is not necessarily because a child is required to tell stories, but because a conversational turn, or an answer to a question, often requires a small narrative contribution. Ninio and Snow (1996) point out that explanations often cannot be differentiated from narratives, since they tend to contain long sequences of language. Oral narratives are an important part of children's daily lives, and the ability to produce narrative discourse is said to be related to learning and academic success. Furthermore, inner dialogue by means of which we explain the world to ourselves may take narrative form.

Background concepts and issues

What is a coherent narrative?

What is a good or a coherent narrative? We seem to instinctively know what is a good story and what is not such a good story. We may say that a good story 'hangs together'; it provides a logical argument; it recounts events accurately and in a viable order; it has a purpose or goal to aim for; it tells us something we did not know previously; or it entertains us. Let us begin by focusing on the concept of coherence and look at a simple definition of it.

Coherence is the interrelateness of ideas (or propositions) so that a listener can make sense of them. This immediately poses two questions: What are ideas or propositions and how do they need to be related to be interpretable by a listener? We will not enter here into a philosophical discussion on the nature of ideas, but will simply accept that we can identify them on the basis of what we know about the world and how we structure our experiences about the world. The latter question we will, however, explore further here. If coherence is the relatedness of ideas, how do the ideas relate, and to what? The following exercise looks at these questions further.

Exercise 5.1

In the following four examples consider what it is that renders the small texts in A acceptable or coherent and the small texts in B (to some degree) unacceptable or incoherent. The best way to work through these examples is to contrast A and B. You need to assume that the texts have been produced by 'fully functioning adults'. On the basis of this exercise, try to provide some more refined definitions of coherence. Think specifically about the following:

How the ideas relate to one another.
How the ideas relate to a(n assumed) topic.
How the ideas develop a topic towards a goal.
How the ideas are sequenced.

Example 1

A: John doesn't get many letters. He doesn't write to anyone.
B: John doesn't get many letters. He painted his house white.

Example 2

The topic for the following two texts is 'How did you come to be in hospital?'

A: It all started about a month ago. I had a pain in my back. Then it got worse and worse. First my doctor told me not to worry about it, but eventually she sent me in here.
B: It all started about a month ago. My dog was being ill and I had to take her to the vet. We are not really an unhealthy family. We eat low-fat spread rather than butter. It's much better for you, I am told.

Example 3

A: I went to Switzerland in March. Switzerland is a beautiful country, but expensive. The Alps are very good for skiing in the spring.
B: I went to Switzerland in March. March is the third month of the year. Years go very quickly. The quickest time I've ever travelled from home to work is 25 minutes.

Example 4

> A: The horse was fed and saddled. I then went for a ride.
> B: I had a nice cup of tea at my neighbour's. She then made it.

Comment 5.1

Before considering each example in turn we need to recognize that when looking at coherence or incoherence we are essentially dealing with probabilistic rather than deterministic phenomena. There are degrees of (in)coherence and these ultimately depend on the interpreter's view of the world and on his/her powers of interpretation (see also Chapter 6). However, what we are attempting to capture in this exercise are some general principles which people seem to operate with when focusing on coherence and not so much on how different individuals may arrive at different interpretations of the same text. These principles will then enable us to say something useful about (in)coherence in children's narratives.

Example 1

Considering A and B side by side, it is the conceptual relationship of 'reason for' which renders the two sentences in A coherent (or related) and a lack of this or any conceptual relationship in B which renders the two sentences in B incoherent (or unrelated). In other words, the second sentence in A (that is, 'He doesn't write to anyone') enables us to infer why John does not get many letters. This inference produces a conceptual relationship between the two sentences (that is, the second sentence is a 'reason for' the first sentence). If you don't write letters to others, others are not likely to write letters to you. With regard to B, however, it is not possible to infer any sensible conceptual relationship between the two sentences, and hence they are perceived as unrelated or incoherent. This is what is meant by relatedness of ideas when we consider coherence in narratives. The (in)ability of the text processor to infer conceptual relationships between ideas in text/discourse renders the text/discourse (in)coherent. Conceptual relationships are the core of coherence. It is worth noting, however, that any subsequent sentences or added context may lead to two apparently unrelated utterances becoming related.

Example 2

This example looks at a more subtle aspect of the concept of coherence. The topic for the two short texts 'How did you come to be in hospital?'

sets up certain expectations as to what ideas to include in the text and how to develop these ideas. Both of the texts express ideas that are related to the topic of illness and hospitals, but the ideas in B do not tell us how and why this person came to be in the hospital. Text A, however, does this very directly, providing an expected order of events as they tend to occur in the world (that is, someone has pain, goes to the doctor, gets worse and ends up in hospital). What this example illustrates, then, is that topics control to a large extent which ideas are expressed in texts and how the ideas are developed towards a goal identified by the topic.

Example 3

The goal-directed nature of coherence is further illustrated by the third set of examples. Contrasting A and B, it is obvious that although in both texts the ideas are related to one another (that is, we can infer conceptual relationships between all the ideas), but in B the ideas are not developed towards any goal and they do not relate directly to any topic. B is an extreme example where there is no global, controlling topic but sentences relate to one another locally, one at a time. This example illustrates the importance of global (or macro) structure in narratives.

Example 4

Texts A and B are used to illustrate how the nature of the world constrains the way in which ideas are presented in texts. It is obviously not possible to drink a cup of tea before it is made, as is depicted in Text B. This is not to say, however, that we cannot talk about events out of the temporal sequence in which they occurred in the world. Indeed, there are grammatical devices enabling us to do just that. We are not suggesting that the utterance 'I made jam with the plums that you brought on Sunday' should be rephrased to reflect the order in which the events occurred (that is, 'You brought some plums on Sunday and then I made some jam out of them'), but rather that some sequences of events are counter to what we know about the world and it is these sequences that need to be expressed in such a way that only the viable interpretation is possible. Texts often, but not invariably, tend to be sequentially structured in the sense that when a topic is developed towards a goal, ideas are mentioned and elaborated one after another, sequentially. In conversations, devices such as 'I forgot to say ...' and 'to go back to an earlier point' indicate that we operate with some notion of a sequential order being part of text coherence. How sequencing relates to different cultural norms and to thinking patterns are other interesting questions.

* * * * * *

This exercise has shown that the concept of coherence has a number of facets to it and that these are describable in more definite terms than perhaps first suggested by the concept of coherence. It has also shown how it is possible to describe *in*coherence in texts by recourse to such basic properties of coherence. Coherence is a person-centred concept, that is, it rests ultimately on people's ability to interpret texts by drawing on their world knowledge and powers of interpretation. But we also suggest that there are some overriding principles that people who produce and interpret narratives follow. We can summarize the general coherence principles highlighted in the above exercise as follows (see also Leinonen-Davies, 1988).

Relational coherence

We perceive a collection of ideas (perhaps expressed in sentences) as having coherence if we can infer conceptual relationships between the ideas. Examples of conceptual relationships would be: X is a reason for Y or X is an elaboration of Y or X is a contradiction of Y (see further de Beaugrande and Dressler, 1981).

This is perceived as 'core coherence' since without the conceptual relatedness we cannot even begin to make decisions about the other aspects of coherence. Without it, we do not have a coherent text, but a collection of unrelated ideas or sentences.

But as we saw in the above exercise, it is not adequate to have ideas which simply relate to one another, the ideas need to be developed towards some goal, and hence the need for the second type of coherence.

Topical coherence

We expect the ideas expressed in a text to relate to a topic and to be developed towards a goal specified by the topic.

Topical coherence attempts to capture the expectations a (perceived) topic sets up about the content of a text and how it should be developed.

Sequential coherence

We expect closely related aspects of the topic to follow one another in sequence or we expect the events in the text to be expressed in such a way that they can be interpreted as reflecting the order of events in the real world. This is not to say that rigid, linear sequencing is always required. If sequential order is disrupted, this can be signalled somehow to the listener.

Let us now see how these somewhat abstract-sounding definitions can be used in thinking about children's difficulties with narrative production.

EXERCISE 5.2

Here is part of a story told by Simon, the same 10-year-old boy already encountered in Chapter 4 (see also Smith and Leinonen, 1992: 261–2). He is telling the story to his speech and language therapist while looking at the story book and while turning the pages as he tells the story. The story has been shared by the two previously. We would ask you to comment on the (in)coherence of this story, by making reference to the above discussion of the three types of coherence.

> John lives with his ... (silence).
> A boy's holding a sheep and there's a dog barking.
> The boy's giving the horse a eat and the boy's holding the horse.
> The man's fishing.
> A dog's barking.
> There's a stream there.
> Some horses near the mountain.
> The boy's holding a hat (saddle) and there's all mans going around sheep.
> All the mans are shouting.
> A boy's going to bed.
> The boy's shouting at the people.
> etc.

Comment 5.2

It is possible to see that the sentences in this story describe various events. These events are illustrated in the book. The events, however, seem not to be connected conceptually to one another (or some are connected very loosely to one another relatively locally). Using the terminology from above, the story can be said to be largely relationally *in*coherent. Relational coherence is the very core of relatedness of ideas, and a lack of relational coherence mounts up to a collection of unrelated sentences. Indeed, Simon's story is not much more than a collection of seemingly unrelated ideas. We say 'seemingly' since this is simply from the text processor's perspective. From Simon's point of view the ideas may possibly connect to a coherent story and he may just have difficulty in expressing them in a way suitable for the listener (although this does not seem likely to us). Our hypothesis is that Simon has difficulty with perceiving the connectedness of (other people's) ideas and when telling a story on the basis of a book he seems to be responding to each picture in turn without regard for a global narrative structure.

Because of this lack of core relatedness (that is, relational incoherence) in Simon's story we cannot begin to say anything about the other two types of coherence. In other words, we cannot have any idea what the topic is, and hence how it could be developed, nor can we say anything about the adequacy of the sequencing of ideas. It is possible that Simon knows what the topic of the story is but has difficulty using the topic in the narrative production in a manner that would render the narrative coherent. He may, of course, have his own theory as to its topic.

Simon's difficulty with narrative production, as reflected by this story, could then be described as a most severe kind, since he did not at this stage manage to relate the ideas to one another in such a way as to enable the listener to compute any useful conceptual relationships between the ideas. As such, he shows difficulty with the very core of narrative production. Indeed, the clinician's opinion was, at that time, that he had only minimal awareness of what stories were. His social behaviour and educational achievements at the time could be seen as consistent with this view.

This exercise has attempted to illustrate how the idea of coherence can help us to specify difficulties with narrative production. Let us consider briefly some further clinical ramifications of the discussion so far.

EXERCISE 5.3

Below are some statements about coherence in narratives and problems with narrative production. Your task is to say whether they are likely to be *true* or *false* and *why*.

(1) Difficulty with relational coherence reflects the most severe difficulty with narrative production.
(2) Difficulty with the understanding of the expectations a topic sets up is likely to result in incoherence in narratives.
(3) Sequencing difficulties have no bearing on narrative production.
(4) Working on the description of pictures in story books would be helpful for developing narrative skills.

Comment 5.3

(1) *True*, in the sense that the very basis of a narrative is the relatedness of ideas to one another. Without such relatedness, expressed in terms of conceptual relationships, no narrative thread exists, but we simply have a collection of unrelated ideas. Such difficulty can be said to be severe from the points of view of both the listener and the person

who is producing the narrative. For the former, (adequate) interpretation is not possible, and for the latter the very core of narrative skill remains to be acquired.

(2) *True*, in that lack of understanding of the topic leads to difficulty in knowing what to include in the narrative (that is, the relevant/salient content) and how to develop the topic towards a goal. Narratives usually have a point to them and they proceed in a certain manner to make this point. Being able to work out what is the topic (which may not be explicitly stated) and then how the topic sets up expectations about the narrative are key skills in narrative (and discourse) production and comprehension.

(3) *False*, in that the production of narratives requires the ability to perceive the sequential nature of events in the world and the ability to structure ideas into a sequence in the narrative itself. But this is not to suggest that a rigid sequence needs to be followed in a narrative.

(4) *False, partly*, in the sense that focus on the description of individual pictures does not promote the relatedness of ideas across pictures and thus does not promote the development of the connectedness of ideas. Children with pragmatic difficulties have been observed to be good at describing the world around them (for example, Leinonen, 1995) but not very good at interrelating these descriptions into a unified whole (for example, Smith and Leinonen, 1992). Having said this, however, we believe that this statement is only partly false, since the very beginnings of narrative development rest on one's ability to observe and describe the world around one, and children with very severe difficulties may need to begin their narrative exploration from such a descriptive basis and from the enjoyment of picture books as objects.

*   *   *   *   *   *

In addition to the kinds of coherence discussed so far, there are several other aspects of narratives which we think are important in the clinical context. We are not in the position to explore them all and have therefore chosen to discuss only one additional area in detail. This area enables us to examine the content of narratives. We would, however, like to refer the reader to Chapter 4 for a discussion on referential usage in narratives and we will return to this discussion in the developmental notes section of this chapter.

Orientation

'Orientation' is an area of narrative work that lends itself to examining how adequate the content of a narrative is. Orientation is a term used in the child language literature on narrative (for example, Peterson, 1990) to describe information relating to the participants, to the place and time of events in narratives, and to the amount of evaluation and explanation of events that has been included. These can be referred to as the 'who', 'where', 'when' and 'why' of the narrative. The events themselves can be referred to as the 'what' of the narrative. In addition to these, narratives tend to have evaluative comments, including reference to emotions/ feelings. When narrating about unique past events and particularly when narrating to a listener unfamiliar with the events, what is clearly important is not only the recounting of the sequence of events which comprise the experience, but also the provision of adequate orientation to the story in terms of who the participants are and how they relate to one another, where and when the events are taking place and why the events occur in the way they do. The ability to provide good orientation to the listener is a long developmental process (see further the 'developmental notes' section below) and rests largely on one's ability to see connections between events, to store and integrate information in a coherent manner, and to assess what the other person needs to know and hence what needs to said and what can be left unsaid. Not only is orientation helpful in a narrative, but the aim is to provide the right amount of orientation.

EXERCISE 5.4

Let us now consider another story from Simon (in addition to 'the boy and the sheep' story which we saw in Exercise 5.2) and examine it in terms of the orientation categories 'what', 'who', 'where', 'when', 'why' and 'evaluation'. In this story Simon is telling of something that happened to him. At the time of telling this he is 12 years old. Your task is to look at each of the orientation categories in turn and to comment on the adequacy of the orientation provided in Simon's story. Simon is telling the story to his speech and language therapist (one of the authors). Compare also this story to 'the boy and the sheep' story and consider whether this kind of exploration suggests anything useful for the clinical management of narrative difficulties.

Simon's Story (dictated to the speech and language therapist):

We are going take some photos down the valley.
Then we walk across and see a house.
It was all like all straw and all breaking.
The wood was all snapping off at the top.
We are going to stay until night.
Then in the afternoon it was going to start to rain so we might as well stay in 'til it brighten up.
Then for a bit we saw it getting darker.
The rain it was really slushing it out.

Then it was starting to all flood in the house and we were going up after and it was breaking.
Then there was all wood flying off the top.
We were frightened.

Comment 5.4

What – This story has narrative continuity. It is possible for the listener to build a picture of what happened and in what order. Thinking back to Simon's 'the boy and the sheep' story, which was simply a description of seemingly unrelated sentences, this story is a great improvement as a coherent unit.

Who – There is no person orientation since Simon uses 'we' from the outset. However, he was asked to narrate about a personal experience and the therapist shares knowledge about his personal background. The person orientation in 'the boy and the sheep' story was inadequate in that it was not possible to say how the characters related to one another and to the events.

Where – There is a fair amount of information about where the events are taking place (for example, in the valley, in the house, the top of the house). This provides the listener with consistent place orientation. In 'the boy and the sheep' story the attempts at place orientation were unsuccessful because of the lack of a global narrative thread.

When – There is some time orientation in the story (for example, after-noon and night). Although it is possible to work out a temporal order of events, this is not always easy because of the confused usage of tense. In Simon's previous story there is no time orientation.

Why – Some cause–effect relationships can be inferred in this story (for example, rain/stay until it brightens up; rain-flood/wood flying). In 'the boy and the sheep' story there is no indication of the reason or motivation for the events and the biggest difference between the two is that in this story the listener can infer conceptual relationships between the ideas whereas this is not possible in the earlier story.

Evaluation – This story has some indication of feelings (for example, 'We were frightened') and description of the mood of the story (for example, 'The rain was slushing it out' or 'It was getting darker'). In 'the boy and the sheep' story there is no evaluation of events or reference to emotions/feelings.

If we compare Simon's narration of 'the boy and the sheep' story book at the age of 10 and this spontaneous telling of a personal experience, we can see that he has come a long way in two years. At the age of 10, Simon had great difficulty with producing narratives which had sufficient continuity and orientation for others to understand them (but see also the section 'personal significance and cooperation' below). Simon was attempting to provide person and place orientation, but this was unsuccessful because there was a total lack of a narrative structure. At the age of 12, however, his story had narrative continuity where conceptual relationships, motivations and reasons were expressed in such a manner that others could follow what was happening. His story also had expressions of mood and feelings, indicating a move away from a simple description towards conveying complete messages to others.

What clinical suggestions might arise from this exploration? At the age of 10, priority would be given to enabling Simon to see connections between and motivations for events (why) and to help him express such basic connectedness (what) adequately for the listener. His attempts at 'who' and 'where' orientation could be later consolidated, particularly emphasizing the importance of others knowing who the participants are and what their roles are. 'When' orientation would not be such a top priority since the temporal sequence of events itself can provide a time reference. Providing 'evaluation' is a developmentally more advanced skill (see 'developmental notes' section below) and given Simon's difficulty with even the very basic features of narratives, this aspect of narratives could be given lower priority. However, it could also be argued that evaluation and personalization of events is what gives the narrative 'the point' and hence it should be encouraged from the outset. Therapy that focuses on adding mood, feelings and evaluation to the basic structure and content of a story moves a narrative further in development.

Personal significance and cooperation

Let us consider one more small narrative from Simon. Simon is here 10 years old (the same age as when he produced 'the boy and the sheep' narrative which we looked at in Exercise 5.2) and he is conversing with his therapist.

> T: Who was in trouble?
> S: Ian and he throwed the hard ball and he hit the window and he smashed the window and he brokened it. He was in the playground and he throwed the hard balled and Mrs (Mr) Jones told our class about it. He took the ball off Ian and he told him off.

This is clearly a coherent narrative with a clear temporal and causal structure, providing an adequate orientation for the listener. How is this possible, given that it would seem from other narratives produced by him at about the same time that he does not know how to integrate information into a coherent narrative? This story differs from the others in two crucial regards: he *initiated it himself* and it describes a relatively small and well-defined event, which Simon *experienced himself*. He was not trying to tell other people's stories, as was the case with the story books. What this would suggest, then, is that Simon is able to piece together information for a specific purpose, but possibly in a much more constrained manner than other 10 year olds. The knowledge that he has the basic ability for narrative production provides a valuable starting point for intervention. The further knowledge that this ability is most readily forthcoming when Simon has something real to tell about his own experiences provides additional guidance for the kind of narrative therapy which may be most facilitative for him. Comparing his personal narratives at ages 10 and 12 suggests that more work on tense usage might have been helpful to Simon and that reassessment using a story book was needed.

It has been noted by many researchers that the context in which activities take place can have an effect on how successfully they are performed, and the above example of Simon's success illustrates this. This example is, however, both contrary to and supportive of what has been suggested in the literature about pragmatically impaired children and their ability to perform context analysis. In their 1991 paper, Bishop and Adams maintain that pragmatically impaired children may have difficulty in analysing the open-ended communicative situation and thus they may be failing more readily in conversations than in more confined test situations. Examples such as the above from Simon would suggest that indeed a well-defined experience in some cases may lead to better narrative production, but there are likely to be other contributing factors such as self-experience and value of events to oneself which enhance narrative production and pragmatic functioning in general.

Underlying abilities

We said in the introductory paragraph that narrative production draws on a multitude of skills, competencies and emotions. Let us consider briefly what these may be and how they connect with the concept of pragmatic impairment. There seem to be three interrelated key skills (or activities) which underlie narrative production.

(1) *Planning and the execution of the plan*: This involves analysing the topic in terms of what expectations it sets up about the content of the narrative and the development of the topic. Some planning is on-line (that is, spontaneous spoken narratives), and hence these are, in

some ways, more demanding than narratives which are preplanned or elicited through pictures/videos.

(2) *Integration of information*: This involves seeing connections between events, characters and phenomena in the world and connecting these for the purpose of communicating a particular message.

(3) *Assessment of the communicative needs of the listener*: This involves decisions about what needs to be explicitly stated and what can be taken as mutually accessible (or mutually known) and hence can be left unsaid.

In addition to these skills, a person has to have something to say. S/he needs to have life experiences and world knowledge, which form the basis for the planning, integration and execution. S/he also needs to have someone s/he wants to communicate with. Problems with any of the above would be reflected in difficulty with narrative production. As we have discussed throughout this book, many pragmatic skills (such as pragmatic comprehension, perceiving relevance in conversation) rest on these kinds of underlying abilities. As we perceive it, they are intrinsically intertwined with pragmatic functioning. So, what manifests on the surface as pragmatic difficulty may have one or more of the above underlying causes. Despite such heterogeneity, the difficulty can still be referred to as being pragmatic in nature in that the manifested difficulties are best described in pragmatic terms.

It is clear that narratives are a rich source of information about various areas of children's functioning. Children's cognitive abilities to plan, integrate and theorize about the world are manifested in their narratives. In Bruner's (1990) terms, narratives are a form of thinking, initiated by human intention and experience. A narrative is also an index of a child's ability to take the processing capacities of the receiver into account and as such reflects his/her development of social cognition. Semantic and syntactic abilities are also manifested in the use of vocabulary and sentence structures in narratives, although it is possible to construct a successful narrative with only rudimentary syntactic and semantic knowledge (see 'developmental notes' section, below).

Methodological issues

A naturally occurring narrative by its very nature is a communicative occurrence. It is fuelled by an experience which one wants to share and an appreciative listener. Bruner (1990) terms this 'reportability'. This poses a dilemma for the researcher or a clinician. How to bring about a situation which is worth reporting on? Questions such as 'What did you do on holiday/on your birthday/at Christmas?' are rather lame attempts at interesting narrative elicitation. Various methodologies have been used successfully in research and clinical practice and we will briefly look at some of them with a view to highlighting their clinical usefulness.

There are basically two ways of eliciting a narrative: generation and retelling. The former is more spontaneous in nature in that the narrative emerges from the child. The generation may, however, be constrained to varying extents by, for instance, picture books or video input. In the clinical context, the child's ability to generate language and discourse spontaneously would decide how spontaneous narrative production can be. Retelling, on the other hand, is constrained by the input to a greater extent and, as such, is affected by one's understanding of the story in the first instance, by one's ability to pay attention and by memory abilities. Generation is clearly a better reflection of a child's internal narrative organization and ability than retelling. It also encourages personal and creative embellishment of events. Retelling can be used to examine how faithful a child is to the original story (see 'clinical data' section, below).

A methodological issue which bears on all narrative production is the effect of the listener on the narrative. Spontaneously produced natural narratives need to consider carefully what the listener knows and what s/he does not. In more controlled elicitation procedures, the listener (the researchers or the clinician) may be sharing the input (for example, the pictures/video) and hence much can be left unsaid, or can be said in a less explicit manner by the child. In these instances, the need to communicate is missing. It is not, however, uncommon in research to bring in a new listener into the elicitation at the point at which the story is to be generated or retold, in this way trying to simulate a more real communicative encounter.

Complexity of the narrative to be retold or generated also affects children's performance, and hence may need to be controlled in both research and the clinical context. A narrative may be complex in terms of its content (for example, unfamiliar content or number of characters) or its structure (for example, events embedded within events). Liles (1993) points out that controlling for complexity is particularly problematic with language-disordered children because of the unavoidable age and experience difference with language-matched controls. What is conceptually about right for the older language-disordered children is too complex for the younger controls, and vice versa.

Research on children's acquisition of narratives has shown that we may not have to worry too much about the method of elicitation, if we are interested in looking at structural properties of narratives. Work by Merritt and Liles (1987, 1989), for instance, has shown that, irrespective of whether stories were generated or retold, children used similar narrative organization. Retelling did, however, render stories longer and more accurate in terms of content. Liles (1993) also makes the point that visual presentation tends to produce more faithful renditions of the original story than audio presentation, in which children's existing world knowledge plays a greater role. Similarly, an unfamiliar listener tends to elicit a greater amount of information from children's stories, primarily inducing greater explicitness of content (predictably) rather than having an effect on the structural organization of the story.

In their work involving children's naturally occurring narratives, Ninio and Snow (1996) have observed that children's narratives are rarely produced as a 'performance' by a child, but are produced cooperatively with the support of others. This support may take the form of getting the story started, clarifying facts, making a psychological perspective explicit (for example, 'that made you really scared') or keeping the story going. One crucial message from this is that in these cooperative activities, a child who finds difficulty getting started, or who struggles with what actually happened and so on, is not seen as failing in any way, but simply as exhibiting normal on-line processing activity. A little help from others has been shown to get the child over the hurdle and on with the story. The communicatively handicapped child may well be a long way from a single narratorship, but capable of constructing a coherent narrative with scaffolding and supporting input from others.

Developmental notes

The development of narrative skill is quite clearly a complex process, given that it is intrinsically intertwined with human cognition, social development, linguistic skill, world knowledge and experience. Yet, it begins as soon as the child has something to tell others and some means (initially non-verbal) of communicating. Nelson (1989) would say that narratives begin to be 'told' in the crib in the form of verbal play. An 18-month-old, who takes an adult's hand, leads him/her to the window, points to a tree where there have been birds previously and says 'gone' is beginning his/her narrative journey. Like in this example, narratives emanate from human experience and human need to share this with others. Without these, narratives cannot begin to be told.

We will aim to overview only some research on children's narrative development and, for a more in-depth review, we refer the reader to Bamberg (1987), McCabe and Peterson (1991) and Liles (1993). We will comment on children's developing knowledge of structural (coherence) properties of narratives and their increasing ability to take the listeners' needs into account (discussed in terms of referential usage and orientation).

Children's early narratives have two main characteristics: they are about the 'here and now' and they are jointly constructed with an adult. One developmental index is, then, the child's move to a single narratorship of the 'there and then'. Children as young as 2 and 3 years of age can recall and discuss past experience truthfully.

EXERCISE 5.5

The following two small 'narratives' are produced by the same 'normally developing' child at the age of 2;2 when playing/conversing with her mother. Each narrative exhibits the child's developing skills, and your task is to say how the narratives come about and also whether one of them could be said to be less/more mature than the other and why. In the transcript 'xxx' denotes unrecognizable utterances.

(1) The mother (M) is playing with the child (C) (Melissa), whose toys are spread around them.

    C: Good. Here's my own little house. I make this steep nice little on top xxx.

        Here's the bright sky. Here's the bright sky.

    M: The bright sky.

    C: Yes. That's the bright sky. I made a bright sky, I have. And the ducks goes river. Ducks is not river.

    M: Isn't it? Not a river.

    C: It is a river. Duck on a river. I make xxx river. Daddy's a river. Making a daddy's a river. Daddy's a river. I making a daddy's and is a castle. Is my castle. I got a new bridge for it.

(2) The mother and the child are pretending to go for a walk to the shops with dolls in a pram which the child is pushing.

    M: Listen. Can we tell them a story on the way to the shops?

    C: Mmm. Story about baby Lucy it.

    M: All right. Now you listen baby 'cause Melissa's going to tell you a story.

    C: xxxx 'bout baby Lucy. Once upon a time little baby Lucy xxx and she went to xxx and see the cows and horses. And she xxx seaside. And see the seaside and the cows and horses and cows and horses and cows.

    M: And horses.

    C: And going seaside.

    M: Mmm

    C: And she had she Mummy and Grandad an Nannies xxxx. And she Daddy and Mummy and Melissa and Katie. Be nice.

Comment 5.5

(1) This 'narrative' is the child's exploration and construction of the current context. The child is verbalizing as she constructs the play scene. She is connecting objects to events (for example, ducks and river; castle and bridge) and as such is showing understanding of relationships in the world. This provides the basis for seeing conceptual relationships in connected narratives. The mother is providing minimal input into the child's construction of the scene, but her comment 'Isn't it? Not a river?' makes a contribution to the child re-evaluating her plan ('It is a river').

(2) Here the child is asked to construct a story and she shows a good understanding of the basic nature of stories. She first tells what the story is about (gives us the topic) and then starts with the well-learned story marker 'Once upon a time ...'. Although she struggles with vocabulary and grammar, she quite clearly understands that stories have activities in which participants engage. She also seems to provide an evaluative comment at the end, 'Be nice', on how nice it is to go to the seaside. This is also a story about past events and an imaginative one in the sense that the child is telling the story as if she were reporting on another person's (that is, Lucy's) experiences. The experiences are more than likely to be her own, but the ability to report them as if they were someone else's shows that she has already had much experience of stories.

It can be said that the second of the narratives demonstrates more maturity than the first, and that a child of just over 2 years of age can already have a good grasp of what a story is. The first of the narratives is a good example of children's beginnings of narrative production, even though this particular child is already capable of going beyond the here and now. What these two small narratives further show is that limited linguistic resources are not an obstacle for demonstrating basic narrative skill.

* * * * * *

Peterson (1990) discusses in her paper how the earliest talk about the past is well supported by routine daily events and is structured around a scaffold provided by familiar adults. First, the majority of content tends to be provided by an adult and the child contributes by minimal yes/no answers. Then, the adult is prompting less, but events are very familiar rather than unique. In the exercise above, the child's narratives seem to reflect the beginnings of this developmental phase. This is also a time when narratives reflect recurrent events in the child's life. Some child language researchers (for example, Nelson, 1986) have described such narratives as script-based. Scripts are structured representations of everyday events, such as going to visit a friend, which may involve getting in a car, getting out of the car, ringing a doorbell, exchanging greetings, playing, having a snack, saying goodbye and so on. The script then provides the structure for the verbal narrative, and a close adherence to the basic events of the script guarantees a coherent outcome. The final outcome of this developmental sequence is for the child to produce narratives of unique past events spontaneously. Children as young as 2 years of age can successfully report on past personal experiences and such narratives constitute a big part of their interactions from about 2-and-a-half onwards (Fivush, Gray and Fromhoff, 1987).

It is not until about the age of 4 that children's narratives begin to have the structure and content which a fully developed narrative needs to have. Although all the components of narratives have started to emerge, the resultant narrative is not by any means an adult equivalent. At this age children will be able to have an introduction, a complication, a resolution and a conclusion in their stories. In such stories the child would first introduce a scene (for example, children are going swimming), in which a complication occurs (for example, one of the children had forgotten to bring his/her swimming costume), which is then resolved (for example, the teacher hires a costume for the child) and so the narrative comes to an end (for example, everyone has a nice time swimming). It is, however, commonly held that it is not until around the age of 6 that children have a narrative structure which has the main component parts of adult narratives. Structural development from thereon involves an increase in the quantity of events included and the complexity of their relationship to one another (for example, events embedded in other events). This development continues well into adolescence.

Peterson's (1990) longitudinal study of the development of 'who', 'when' and 'where' orientation to unfamiliar adults by 10 children between the ages of 2;0 and 3;6 indicated that 'who' orientation was the least developed in the age period. The children used pronouns and proper names, for instance, without specifying to the listener who the referents were. This suggests that adequate person orientation would not begin to develop until after the age of 3;6. 'When', or time, orientation was almost non-existent at first, but began to emerge during the study. 'Where', or place orientation, was common from the beginning and showed steady improvement with age. So, by about the age of 4 children can already provide some orientation as to who the participants are and where and when the events take place but this development continues through the school years. Bamberg and Damrad-Frye's (1991) analysis of 5–9-year-old children's and adults' usage of evaluative comments showed that, compared with adults, children in this age range used such comments in a more local manner ('X is happy') rather than in a more global manner ('Everyone seemed happy'). This was interpreted to reflect the adults' appreciation of a more global or macro-level of the story as opposed to the children's more local focus.

Further research into children's developing abilities of referential usage by Bennett-Kastor (1983) (see also, Bamberg, 1987) has suggested that children as young as 2 are able to use noun phrases and pronouns in successive clauses cohesively, but that it is not until around the age of 5 that they can show better command of using pronouns coherently in extended narratives with several characters (see also Chapter 4). Looking at the many aspects of narrative production together, the age of 5 seems to be when there is an accelerated development in narrative skill. Liles (1993) suggests that the understanding of the global narrative structure seems to begin to accelerate at this age. But, as the work of Bamberg and Damrad-Frye (1991) shows, even 9-year-olds have not yet reached the adult command of particular evaluative devices which reflect global discourse organization.

Clinical populations

The question of whether language disorder has an effect on children's ability to produce coherent and cohesive narratives is one that has been discussed particularly by Liles and colleagues (Liles, 1985, 1987, 1993; Merritt and Liles, 1987, 1989; Purcell and Liles, 1992). Liles (1985) analysed spoken narratives produced by 20 normal and language-disordered children (aged 7;6 to 10;6) using Halliday and Hasan's cohesion categories which enable one to examine how utterances are connected in discourse. She found that the two groups differed in the way that they organized cohesion in their narratives and in terms of how adequate their cohesive ties were. For instance, the language-disordered group used fewer personal pronouns to link sentences together. As Liles points out, the use of such pronouns results in a complex chaining of ideas as the ties distribute throughout the narrative and the language-disordered children seemed to have difficulty with such chaining. Interestingly, however, the groups performed very similarly when telling the story to a listener who knew the story and when telling it to an uninformed listener. Both groups used many more incomplete ties with the informed listener as compared with the uninformed listener. This indicates similar difficulty with adjusting the story to the needs of the listener.

In another study, using the same children as above, Liles (1987) examined the children's ability to produce adequate story episodes. An episode can be described as a larger component of meaning in a narrative. Episodes, such as 'event initiations', 'plans', 'attempts at reaching goals' and 'resolutions of conflict', can be said to be in global hierarchical relationships to one another. These relationships are considered global (or logical) in that they are not dependent on the specific content of the narrative (see also 'conceptual relationships' in the background section, above). Episodes may be, for instance, in a temporal or a causal relationship to one another. Narrators tend to make such relationships explicit by using conjunctions such as 'then', 'so' and 'therefore'. Given the global rather than local nature of episodes, they can be regarded as reflecting some macro-level cognitive structures. Within this background, Liles discovered that both groups of children found the signalling of conjunctive relations across episode boundaries more difficult than elsewhere in discourse. This is interpreted as reflecting the increased cognitive complexity involved when processing at these macro-level boundaries as opposed to more local processing within discourse. It is further suggested that the difficulty for a subset of the language-disordered group was a likely reflection of their poor initial understanding of how the episodes in the story were related. It was found that when the children's comprehension of the story was checked, the language-disordered children had more difficulty in answering questions that focused on relational aspects of the story in comparison with questions that checked factual information. Even though both groups were poor at episode boundaries, across-group comparison of inaccurate conjunctive ties showed that the language-disordered children produced a greater number of inaccurate conjunctions regardless of the episode organization. This shows general difficulty with cohesive signalling. One of the most striking differences in this study was, however, that the normal children added episode units, thus providing more information, for an uninformed listener whereas the language-disordered group did not. Liles argues that this is a reflection of the children's inability to produce more complex stories rather than of their inability to recognize the need to provide further information.

These specific findings seem to suggest that at least some language-disordered children are likely to experience difficulty with discourse organization and with the signalling of semantic connectedness across sentences. Liles (1993) suggests that one way forward is to examine the extent to which such difficulties are a reflection of linguistic, cognitive or social difficulties. She suggests that one possibility is that there may be language-disordered children who have sufficient language to demonstrate a command of more local narrative structures (for example, intersentential cohesion) but the language command may not be sufficient for the signalling of cognitively more complex connections at a macro-level of organization. These kinds of questions remain to be investigated. There is also a real need to establish a reliable measure of the various aspects of narrative ability which could be used in clinical assessment procedures.

Even though there are only a few direct references in the literature to pragmatically impaired children as narrators (for example, Smith and Leinonen, 1992), work on such children's pragmatic functioning would enable one to predict difficulties with narrative construction. The case studies of McTear (1985b) and Conti-Ramsden and Gunn (1986) report on their subjects' difficulties with verbal reasoning. The reported difficulties with making inferences and predictions about a simple course of action, for instance, would predict problems with narrative construction. Similarly, Leinonen and Letts' (1997b) case study of a pragmatically impaired girl reported particular difficulty in answering questions that placed heavy inferential demands on the child. Bishop and Adams' (1989) observations of pragmatically impaired children's tendency to provide too much or too little information (for example, referential usage) and their difficulty with topic maintenance are likely to be manifest in the narrative mode, too. So, narrative production is likely to be problematic to children with pragmatic difficulties since it rests on the ability to make connections, to provide adequate information to the listener and to maintain a topic over a period of time. Given also that explanations offered for questions often include narrative sequences (Ninio and Snow, 1996), the children's conversational difficulties may also have a narrative component. Children's ability to explain the world to themselves may similarly be affected by difficulty with narrative construction.

In spite of the paucity of narrative studies of pragmatically impaired children, the clinical value of narratives has been recognized throughout the literature. In the Conti-Ramsden and Gunn study (1986) the therapy programme included the use of stories to encourage the child to work out logical links between events. Smith and Leinonen (1992) make frequent reference to the therapeutic importance of narratives and illustrate this by using clinical data. Bishop and Edmundson (1987) found performance on the Bus Story (Renfrew, 1969) to be a good predictor of whether or not a child's language difficulties would resolve by the age of 5;6. In the Bus Story test a child has to retell a story which accompanies pictures and the child's story is scored for accuracy of information given and for the average number of words in the five longest sentences. Smedley's (1989) suggestions of how to use written work in therapy with pragmatically impaired children incorporates work on seeing temporal connections through descriptions of what is happening in the classroom and understanding of causal relationships in written stories. A detailed case study by Klecan-Aker (1993) of a boy (aged 8;8) with language/learning difficulties looked at the effects of a treatment programme on his story-telling abilities. This work emphasizes the close link between story telling and academic success, and hence the importance of narration in therapy, so that the child could take part in the full range of classroom activities. The treatment programme consisted of teaching the child about overall story organization and coherence (for example, the child was told that telling stories was like baking a cake. One needed a recipe, or an overall plan, which needed to be followed in the right order). Focus was also on helping the child to see conceptual relationships between events, such as cause and effect. The child was to choose multiple-choice answers to 'why' questions after hearing short stories.

It is apparent from these few small studies that therapists have long known the value of working with narratives when working with children who have pragmatic difficulties. What remains to be done is for researchers to investigate what children with pragmatic problems are like as narrators. This research would then lend further support to the validity of story telling as a therapeutic tool with communicatively impaired children.

Clinical data

We will now examine many of the points made so far by considering narrative data from one child with pragmatic and to a much lesser degree linguistic difficulties. These data come from a retelling task.

EXERCISE 5.6

In the following data sample Sarah, aged 9;8, is retelling a story to one of the authors. These data are from a study by Leinonen, Letts and Parke (1994). The adult tells Sarah that she is going to hear a story which goes with a cartoon of eight pictures. The story and the pictures are from Fletcher and Birt (1983). Sarah is told to listen very carefully and to look at the pictures at the same time as the story is being told. She is also told beforehand that she will be asked to tell the story back after the adult has finished telling it. Here is first the story as told by the adult (P1, P2 and so on indicate how the text relates to the pictures) and then Sarah's retelling of the story.

Input story

Mr Smith phones Mr Plummer to invite him and his wife for dinner on Friday at 8 o'clock (P1). Mr and Mrs Smith spend all afternoon cooking. They prepare a whole salmon for the main dish (P2). The table is laid and the salmon is put in its place and no one notices the cat under the table (P3). Mr and Mrs Smith go upstairs to get ready for the dinner party (P4). At 8 o'clock the Plummers arrive. Mrs Plummer has some flowers with her (P5). They go into the dining room to start dinner (a loud intake of breath from the adult telling the story). The salmon has gone. 'Oh dear' says Mrs Smith 'What can we do?' (P6). Mr Smith dashes out to the fish and chip shop (P7). Everyone enjoys their unexpected dinner, especially the cat (P8).

Sarah's retelling of the input story

A: OK? Now you tell me the story [starting from the beginning]

S: [eeh – unintelligible] (mumbled) tell that—ehh (unintelligible) Mr Smith (Sarah looks at all the pictures and points to them)

A: OK. You just start telling from the top.

S: eeh——I don't know what to say.

A: Have a look at the pictures.

S: Oh yeah. This is Friday. This is Friday dinner. (Sarah points to P1 where Mr Plummer is talking on the phone to Mr Smith and is writing '8 pm Friday dinner with Smiths' on a notepad.)

A: Yes. The man is writing something (A misunderstands S since she mumbles). Speak nice and clear.

S: Mmmmm——

A: What's happened. What is happening here? (A points to P1.)

S: eeeeh—Mr Smith is washing up (this is depicted in P2). And there is a big salmon. And—Mr Smith put the—and (unintelligible) the candlelight on top of the candles (in P3 the salmon is on the table, the cat under the table and Mr Smith lighting candles on the table). And there's wine. And Mr and Mrs Smith got ready for the dinner party. And—I don't know these people's names (S points to the Plummers in P5).

A: Do you want to invent them names. Give them some names.

S: Eeeh——

A: Mr and Mrs (rising intonation)

S: Eeeh—

A: Brown. Call them Brown.

S: Mr and Mrs Brown came to the tea party. Mrs Brown brought some flowers. And Mr Smith and Mrs Smith and Mr Brown and Mrs Brown saw the salmon and it gone (laughter). Mr Smith ran out and went to the fish and chip shop. And—And they—And Mr Smith and Mrs Smith. Mr Brown Mrs Brown. No. Mrs Brown and Mr Brown 'n' Mr Smith and Mrs Smith had a lovely dinner party.

A: Yes—Have you finished?

S: Yeah

(End of story but the conversation carried on as follows)

A: OK. Thank you. What do you think the cat did?

S: Licking (S points to P8 where the cat is licking its paws next to the table).

A: Yes. Licking. But what do you think the cat did (emphasis on the word did).

S: Eating the salmon.

A: The cat ate the salmon.

S: Yeah.

A: So, is that why they could not eat the salmon themselves?

S: No.

A: All right, but why do you think they went to the fish and chip shop?

S: Eeeh—because the salmon—because the salmon was gone so so the cat
    was eating it.
A: Yeah. So there was nothing left for them to eat.
S: No (laughter).
A: So they had to go 'n' get fish and chips.
S: (laughter)

On the basis of this data sample, your task is now to comment on the narrative produced by Sarah. Refer back to the categories 'what', 'who', 'where', 'when', 'why' and 'evaluation', which were discussed in the background section.

(A) When commenting on the 'what' check for inclusion of the basic events as follows: (1) invitation; (2) preparation of dinner; (3) put salmon on table; (4) don't see cat; (5) P's arrival; (6) salmon gone; (7) what can be done?; (8) fish and chip shop; (9) all enjoy dinner. Lexical identity is not required here. Credit Sarah with the key feature if the idea is expressed, using whatever words.

(B) When commenting on the 'who', or person orientation, note particularly the use of proper names, pronouns and other proforms and the role of the cat in the story and how this is handled. There are 10 instances of proper nouns and nine instances of pronouns and other proforms in the input story.

(C) When focusing on the 'when', or time orientation, pay attention to temporal order. There are four references to time in the input text.

(D) When discussing the 'where', or place orientation, note that there are five explicit place adverbials in the input text.

(E) 'Why' refers to the conceptual relationships in the story. There are reasons for the story events. For instance, Mr Smith phones Mr Plummer with a view to issuing an invitation. Or Mr Smith has to go to the fish and chip shop because the cat ate the salmon. And the cat was able to eat the salmon because it sneaked under the table. When discussing 'why' consider how well Sarah signals to the listener these kinds of key relationships.

(F) For 'evaluation' comment on how mood and feelings of characters and events are dealt with. There are certain words and phrases in the input text which indicate mood and feelings in the story: the Smiths 'spend all afternoon cooking'; the gasp from the adult telling the story when they enter the dining room; the words uttered by Mrs Smith when the salmon's disappearance is discovered; Mr Smith 'dashes out to the fish and chip shop'; the dinner being enjoyed by all; the dinner being enjoyed especially by the cat.

Comment 5.6

The task has also been carried out with five linguistically normally functioning children (range 8;5–11;2; Sarah was 9;8) and its content and structure seemed suitable for this age range (discussion in Leinonen, Letts and Parke, 1994). Let us begin with some general comments about Sarah's retelling of the story.

She has great difficulty getting started. It is not clear whether this is because she has not understood what is expected of her or because she does not know what a story is and how to tell one. It is not likely that she would not have access to the linguistic resources needed for the story as her linguistic functioning in terms of grammar and word knowledge are considered near age appropriate (details in Leinonen and Letts, 1997b). From what she tells and what we can infer from the conversation in the end, she has understood the basic ideas in the story and hence should be able to retell them, given particularly that she has the pictures to aid memory. She eventually begins her story by reading what is written on Mr Plummer's notepad in the first picture. She then proceeds to describe certain aspects of the next two pictures (that is, Mr Smith washing up and lighting candles; and there is wine). In other words, she is not attempting to retell the input story at this point, but simply describes what she sees in the pictures. It is not until she refers to Mr and Mrs Smith getting ready for the dinner party that she starts to follow the story as it was originally told. There is a possibility that the pictures from here onwards more explicitly depict the events in the story and that Sarah may still be relying heavily on the pictures rather than the input story.

Let us now consider how the 'what', 'who', 'where', 'when', 'why' and 'evaluation' are signalled in Sarah's story.

What: Sarah mentions five out of the nine key features or events. She mentions that there is a big salmon, that the Plummers (renamed as the Browns) arrive, that the salmon is gone from the table, that Mr Smith goes to a fish and chip shop and that all have a lovely dinner party. In the Leinonen, Letts and Parke (1994) study, the five control children mentioned between seven and eight of the key features. In addition, Sarah mentions from the input story that Mrs Plummer brings some flowers (these can also be seen in the picture).

Who: The characters are fairly straightforward in this story in terms of how they relate to one another. Sarah becomes quite fixated on the characters' names after she struggles with Mr and Mrs Plummer's names. The input text has 10 instances of proper names and nine pronouns and other proforms. Sarah uses only two instances of a pronoun (one of them an abandoned attempt at 'they'), no other proforms and 21 proper nouns. In the course of a narrative one would expect a narrator to use proforms, once characters have been introduced. This did not happen with Sarah. Interestingly, the cat is not mentioned at all by her. However, in the conversation following the story, it is clear that Sarah had understood that the cat ate the salmon. The adult asks two questions as an attempt to probe Sarah's understanding of the role of the cat ('But what do you think the cat did?' and 'But why do you think they went to the fish and chip shop?') and Sarah's answers to both of these questions showed that she knew what the cat had done and what the consequences of this action were for the dinner party.

When: Sarah expresses the temporal order of events in the story adequately. This may simply be a reflection of the order of the pictures. She does not use any other time references except the word 'Friday' in the beginning (which was the day the party was to take place) and this was not mentioned in the input story. Sarah read the word 'Friday' in the first picture.

Where: Place in this story has a reasonably significant role in that the salmon was on the table and the cat under the same table, which then sets up the possibility for the salmon being eaten by the cat. This is not expressed in Sarah's story. Sarah does express the going to the fish and chip shop explicitly, and in the conversation that followed she showed some understanding of the significance of Mr Smith going there. The other place references in the input story are supportive of the plot, and again they are all ignored in Sarah's story.

Why: Sarah does not make any conceptual relationships explicit in her story. Largely because we know the input text we are able to link her seemingly unconnected descriptions to one another. There are lexical links such as 'washing up - cooking - salmon - wine - dinner party etc.' which signal semantic connectedness across utterances. There is one odd expression which on the surface would indicate an impossible relationship in the world ('...saw the salmon and it was gone'). This may, of course, reflect an expressive language problem.

Evaluation: Sarah's story has two expressions which indicate mood: 'Mr Smith ran out...' can be seen as indicating some urgency, and 'lovely dinner party' reflects everyone's enjoyment of the dinner.

Linguistic interpretation

Retelling task: accuracy and completeness

In the background section we considered retelling and generation as two means of eliciting stories and we noted that the former is more limited in terms of how much it tells about a child's internal organization of narrative structure. This may well be true, but tasks, such as the one carried out with Sarah, have their value in enabling one to check for the child's comprehension of narrative structure, his/her ability to tell other people's stories, his/her concern for accuracy and faithfulness to the original story, and they also give a view of possible memory difficulties. Leinonen, Letts and Parke (1994) noted that on the same Dinner Party task, the five control children showed remarkable convergence on the main points of the story. The absence of a real communicative impulse (the researcher obviously knew the story) led the children to be very faithful to the input text rather than providing a more creative account of the given story. The children seemed to know exactly what was expected of them. They seemed to assume that criteria such as completeness and accuracy were important and their performance seemed to be predicated on their knowledge of what a narrative is. Sarah, however, seems much less confident in her knowledge of what the task requires of her. Her story suggests that she may be uncertain of how a narrative is structured and further that she was not aiming for completeness and accuracy.

Leinonen, Letts and Parke (1994) further suggest that the control children seemed to operate as if there were five principles to observe in this task: (1) include the salient (key) points; (2) adhere to the order of input (reinforced by the pictures); (3) include much of the input vocabulary and vary it within strict limits; (4) add (practically) nothing; (5) choose a time reference and stick to it. If we consider Sarah's performance in relation to these five principles, we can see that she does not follow them to any great degree (for whatever reason). She does not include all the salient points and she includes non-salient and non-mentioned information (for example, the candlelight on top of the candles). She is not faithful to the input vocabulary, but is faithful to the order of events. The pictures are likely to be playing a role in the latter. Her time reference is consistent.

Underlying abilities

Data exploration, such as presented here, does not aim to explain why any of the observed patterns occur and further research is required to this end. Meanwhile, Leinonen, Letts and Parke (1994) discuss some abilities that are likely to come into play in a recall task such as the one used with Sarah:

(A) The ability to understand the task and, perhaps, to see the point of it.

(B) The ability to understand how the ideas in the input text relate to an assumed topic (macro level) and to one another (micro level).

(C) The ability to remember the ideas expressed in the input text.
(D) The ability to reanalyse and internalize the text within the confines of
      the input text.
(E) The ability to relate the text to the pictures (to integrate the visual and
      lexical information).
(F) The ability to process the input text with the required speed.

Given Sarah's story, we can make some guesses as to which of these
areas may be relevant to her difficulties. She may not have understood
what the task was when it was explained to her and hence may not have
listened to the story with a view to retelling. She had difficulty starting the
retelling and it was not until the pictures became more explicit in their
relationship to the input story that she seemed to converge with the
input. The possibility that she did not understand the story, at either a
macro or a micro level, is perhaps not likely, given the conversation at the
end of the story. It seems that she was aware of the main point of the story
and how the other events related to this (that is, that the cat ate the
salmon intended for the dinner party and hence the need to buy fish and
chips). An inability to remember the story (as opposed to understand it) is
another possibility. She was not faithful to the input story, in terms of lexis
and expression (as were the controls). Difficulty involved in reanalysing
the story with a view to knowing what is salient to include in the retelling
of it is another possibility but there is no way of knowing from the data
whether this is a problem for Sarah. Nor can we know whether she was
not able to integrate the story with the pictures and, hence, the retelling
of it on the basis of the pictures would cause problems.

Description

It has been observed in research that pragmatically impaired children tend
to be good at describing the world around them, as they observe it (for
example, Leinonen, 1995; Leinonen and Letts, 1997b) (although they may
differ from normally functioning children in what they regard as salient).
Description is immediate and concrete, whereas story telling and reporting
are often neither, and also sometimes imaginary. Sarah's retelling of the
story seems to be very reliant on the immediately observable (that is, the
pictures). Her initial struggles with beginning the retelling are resolved by
describing some non-mentioned aspect of the first few pictures. It may also
be that the adult's attempts at getting Sarah going are in fact interpreted by
Sarah as instructions for picture descriptions ('You start telling from the
top', 'Have a look at the pictures', 'What is happening here?'). When
describing, a child need not be concerned with the communicative
demands of the situation (that is, who the speaker is, what effect his utter-

ance may have, and so on) and hence for children who have particular problems with communicating in an open-ended context, description of the world as it is observed is a much less taxing way of honouring one's communicative obligation of saying something. It is also worth noting that it is not uncommon for children with pragmatic difficulties to tell fairly complex stories as if they were true when in fact it is known to the listener that the content of the story is largely fictional (or may be found to be so at a later date). We may query whether this reflects some difficulty on the child's part to know what a story is for.

Orientation

We explored Sarah's retelling in terms of the categories 'what', 'who', 'where', 'when', 'why' and 'evaluation'. The 'what' enables us to say something about the core coherence of the narrative in terms of how events in the story are reported and sequenced. Sarah's story was more limited in terms of what was mentioned when compared with the control data in Leinonen, Letts and Parke (1994). The cat and its antics were not mentioned by Sarah at all, nor did she make the implicit role of the cat explicit. The control children did not make the cat's role explicit either. They probably followed the example of the input text. It is more difficult to know whether this was the case with Sarah, since she in general was not faithful to the input text. Yet, this may be the case since, as the conversation after the story telling shows, she did understand the role of the cat in the events. With regard to 'who' orientation, we noted that Sarah used proper names rather than pronouns. The use of pronouns requires a good command of the input story in order for one to be able to relate pronouns with their antecedents appropriately. The use of proper names is almost as if Sarah were concerned that all the participants were correctly and completely identified without any possible confusion. Another possibility is, of course, that she does not know when it is appropriate to use pronouns, and hence relies on the proper noun strategy. As for 'when' and 'where' orientation, Sarah seems to follow the temporal order of events reasonably, but she has only minimal expression of place orientation (that is, fish and chip shop). Three out of the five control children explicitly stated that the cat was under the table. Place and time expressions are not paramount for maintaining core coherence and Sarah's ignoring them may reflect her attempt at simply getting the basic story retold. When struggling with detail (be it for memory or other reasons, see (2) above), a useful strategy is to keep strictly to the minimum which will still preserve the overall goal (that is, telling a story). One of the problems in Sarah's story is that conceptual relationships (that is, 'why') are not made explicit. Despite this, the story still (just about) hangs together for the listener. The point is, however, that this is dependent more on the listener's powers of providing the story than on Sarah making it clear on the surface how the story should be interpreted. 'Evaluation' is not strongly present in Sarah's story and the surprise in the input text, when the disappearance of the salmon is discovered, is not recorded at all. Overall, then, Sarah manages to reproduce some basic events in the story which then enable the listener to piece together an account of what was likely to have happened. What is missing, however, is an explicit account of some key features of the story and most of the finer, background, detail mentioned in the input text.

Clinical interpretation

It is clear from what has been said already that the ability to tell stories depends on a multitude of pragmatic and other skills and we should not be surprised that children with pragmatic impairments have difficulty in this area. It is also highly likely that children with any degree of language impairment will have difficulty with narratives, and this will go some way towards explaining the diagnostic value attributed to the information section of the Bus Story test (Renfrew, 1969) by Bishop and Edmundson (1987). At the same time, story telling and exposition in general are important skills in the classroom (and mentioned explicitly in the National Curriculum in the UK), and the child needs to be able to demonstrate these both in speaking and in writing. Giving the child the opportunity to develop narrative skills in the clinical situation has obvious value.

To unpick Sarah's problems, as shown in the above extract, the first problem is that she is unclear as to the key components and structure of 'a story'. As a result, she cannot get started with the retell task, even though the story itself has already been given to her. Explicit practice in working through the main parts of a story is necessary, perhaps initially by identifying these parts for her and asking her to answer explicit questions – for example, 'who' are the main characters; 'where' did this take place; 'what' happens; do we need to say anything about 'when'; was it a happy/funny/sad story ('evaluation')? The story itself could be presented either in the popular picture sequence format, or perhaps as a retell task. With picture sequences, care needs to be taken that the child understands that the pictures link together to form a story and that the child does not merely talk about each picture in turn. It may be helpful to remove the pictures from view for this exercise, but allow the child to refer back to them where necessary if s/he cannot remember what happens. Length and complexity of the stories can be increased as the child becomes more competent at this. Better still than either picture sequences or retell exercises are interesting story books that do not contain any written words. If written text is also present, the child may be distracted by this and try to read the story. In the 'Dinner Party' task, Sarah started to read the only written information (on a notepad next to the phone) available in the pictures when she was struggling to get started. We can, of course, view this as a positive strategy, too, and one which can be used in narrative-based therapy.

The next step would be to help the child to work out for him/herself what the key components of the story are, without relying on a set of questions. Finally, the child would be encouraged to tell his or her own stories. Given the problems that some pragmatically impaired children may have with confabulation, some discussion of truth versus fiction might be appropriate here, and how to indicate that a story is fiction as opposed to something that really happened.

When a child has a firm grasp of the key components that go to make up a story, s/he may be able to tell the story in a vivid and entertaining manner even if skills at other linguistic levels are lacking. The story may be expressed using key words in simple or telegraphic sentences, or even by means of gestures and vocalization. However, in situations where more standard language forms are required (and where the child has the potential to develop these), the ability to use referring expressions (see Chapter 4) such as pronouns appropriately will be important. If the child is old enough to access the written form, specific structural exercises linking pronouns and other deictic words to their referents may be of value. The child could then analyse his or her own narratives in the same way. For Sarah, it may be premature at this stage to work on this area, since so many aspects of her story telling are problematic; one can see, however, that it would be possible to go through some of her use of proper names, establish whether the person or persons have already been mentioned and identified, and then discuss which pronouns might suitably replace these names.

Summary

We have hoped to demonstrate in this chapter that narrative production is a multifaceted skill which children start to acquire very early and which continues to develop through the school years. We have discussed the kinds of features a coherent narrative needs to have in order for it to function as a narrative. We came to the conclusion that the ability to perceive conceptual relationships in the world and the ability to represent these in a narrative in a manner that makes interpretation possible for others are the core abilities required in narrative production. The ability to analyse topics with a view to identifying the expectations they set up about both the structure and the content of the narrative is also an important skill associated with narrative production. We also made the point that conversational contributions, including giving explanations, involve narrative ability and hence narratives are an important part of children's lives. Given this, it is not surprising that narrative ability is said to correlate with academic success. Children who have pragmatic difficulties may well have problems at some stage of their development with the production of narratives, given that the underlying skills necessary for narrative production overlap with skills needed for other forms of pragmatic functioning.

Chapter 6: Comprehension of pragmatic meaning

Key words: linguistic comprehension, pragmatic comprehension, descriptive meaning, inferential meaning, inferencing, pragmatic demands of input questions, intermittency of problematic behaviours.

Aims

Comprehension difficulty has been a somewhat neglected area of research among specifically language impaired children (SLI) and children with pragmatic difficulties. The literature on children's pragmatic impairments is beginning to recognize that in order to move on from descriptive accounts of surface behaviours, we need to begin to consider children's functioning in areas which may underpin (un)successful communication. To this end, suggestions have highlighted the importance of comprehension in successful communication and the role of cognitive skills such as inferencing in making sense of language input, the communicative behaviour of others and the world in general. This chapter aims to explore the following:

Key questions:
What is comprehension and what can affect it?
What is linguistic comprehension?
What is pragmatic comprehension?
What is inferencing and how does it relate to comprehension?
What are language-disordered children like as comprehenders?
What are pragmatically impaired children like as comprehenders?
Why is comprehension important for understanding pragmatic impairment?
Can different types of input question have an effect on pragmatic performance?
What clinical implications must we consider?

It will be shown that exploration of these topics yields valuable insight into the nature of some children's pragmatic difficulties by pinpointing very specific problem areas, leading to more targeted intervention suggestions. It will also be highlighted that the same surface communicative behaviours can have varying underlying explanations. Bishop (1997) provides a comprehensive overview of the development of comprehension in normal and disordered populations.

Background concepts and issues

What is comprehension? It is perhaps needless to say that there is no clear answer to this question. There are simply some issues and controversies that need to be borne in mind when focusing on children's (in)ability to comprehend language and connected discourse. It is common to differentiate between linguistic (syntactic/semantic) comprehension and comprehension at the discourse and pragmatic levels. What are the differences?

Linguistic comprehension

You may be familiar with the following situations:

(1) Imagine that you overhear the following utterance of some other people's conversation.

That kind of experimenting is very dangerous.

It is possible to understand every word in this utterance, but it is not possible to really know what it is about or what its significance is. As we do not know the context in which this utterance is produced, we cannot agree or disagree with what has been said. It is not possible to say whether the content of the utterance is true or false.
(2) Most of us have been in a situation in which we can identify the topic, but, even so, the full meaning of what has been said remains obscure. For example, many people have had the experience of trying to understand a book or a lecture on a topic that is so unfamiliar that even though the words and sentences are comprehensible, it is not possible to appreciate the import of what has been read or heard.

In both of these examples, we can be said to have comprehended linguistically, but not pragmatically. Linguistic comprehension can be said to involve understanding word meanings (level of semantics) and how a combination of words according to the grammar of the language produces a sentence meaning (level of syntax).

EXERCISE 6.1

Consider the following four examples and explore: (1) whether you can say if the sentences are true or false in the world (or whether you agree or disagree with what is being said) and, if not, why not; (2) whether you have comprehended anything and what contributions words and grammar make to your comprehension

(A) 'In order to operate the feeder, the ground bar must be lowered into the slant position and the pin must be rotated. This will free the feeder arm.'
(B) 'Violins are playing songs on my spinal cord.'
(C) 'Why don't you slam the door?'
(D) 'The task is quite time consuming. It is also labour intensive. It cannot be guaranteed that a week and five people is adequate for completion.'

Comment 6.1

(1) It is not possible to say whether the sentences are true or false, because we do not know the contexts in which they occur. We may be able to construct possible contexts for (A), (C) and (D), at least, and make truth judgements on the basis of these contexts, but these contexts may not have been the original ones. For instance, (C) might have been uttered in at least the following two contexts, giving rise to very different meanings for the sentence:
Context 1: Two people are trying to close a car door, which is jammed. In this context the utterance functions as a suggestion.
Context 2: Two people share a car regularly, and the driver always slams the door when getting out of the car, which the passenger does not appreciate and thus utters (C). In this context, the utterance is ironical and has the opposite meaning – 'Please do not slam the door'.
(2) We can comprehend all the sentences linguistically and we can make some connections between the sentences in the texts. For (A), (C) and (D), comprehension is based on both word meaning and syntax, whereas for (B) we 'comprehend' syntactically alone. For (B) we can see that there are objects and an event which relate to one another in certain ways (that is, X is doing Y with Z). It is our knowledge of

grammar that enables us to attribute this minimal meaning for the sentence. If a language-disordered person had produced this sentence, we could say that the person is functioning adequately at a basic grammatical level, and the problem would lie with choice of appropriate words to fill the grammatical slots.

*   *   *   *   *   *

This exercise has shown that it is possible to work out some meaning on the basis of the linguistic expression alone (words and grammar), but that such 'comprehension' is very limited. We need to be able to construct a context mentally in which sentences and texts occur in order to understand them fully – in order to understand their significance.

Pragmatic comprehension

What kind of meaning is there beyond linguistically signalled meaning? There is meaning that is found in the context and meaning that is worked out on the basis of our knowledge of the world. Let us consider some examples:

(A) '*He* is married to *her* not *her*' (speaker is nodding in the appropriate directions) – the meanings of the pronouns are found in *the physical context*.

(B) 'My mother is delighted about the new cooker. *She* thinks that *it* is much better than the old one' – the meanings of the pronouns are found in *the verbal context*.

(C) 'My husband did a good job with our fireplace' – depending on the intentions of the speaker this may indicate admiration, boasting, irony, belittling, persuasion. This kind of additional meaning can be referred to as *speech act meaning* (see further Chapter 2).

(D) 'It's water under the bridge' – depending on the context and intentions of the speaker this may mean 'Let's forget all about what has happened' or 'It's water under the bridge, not oil'. The former refers to *non-literal meaning* and the latter to *literal meaning*.

(E) Mary went to buy an ice-cream. She had left her money at home. 'Never mind' said the shopkeeper 'You can pay next time'. Even though it is not explicitly (linguistically) stated, we can work out *the implied meaning* that Mary got her ice-cream.

(F) 'The film was very frightening' – the definite expression in front of 'film' means that the speaker assumes this information is shared by him/her and the listener. The expression *presupposes* this information.

(G) 'I managed to tell him the bad news' – the word 'manage' *implies* that the speaker found the telling of the bad news difficult for some reason.

(H) 'You will feel better soon' – this has a different *personal meaning or significance* for a bereaved person and a person who has suddenly felt slightly faint.

These are all instances where the language expression itself does not provide the full meaning of the expression, but listeners need to 'go elsewhere' (into the context or their world knowledge) to comprehend the message. We can be said to be comprehending pragmatically, when we go beyond the language expression.

Austin (1962) was one of the first to alert people to intended speaker meaning in communication (see also Chapter 2). When comprehending utterances, the listener's task is to work out the intentions and beliefs the speaker holds when speaking. In the expression 'I promise to beat you up' the linguistic expression is not a reliable clue to the intended meaning. As Searle (1969) states, one of the conditions for a promise is that the speaker believes that the listener wants the act to be performed. According to this criterion the above expression would function as a threat rather than as a promise. The important point is that it is the intentions and beliefs of the speaker which endow an utterance with speech act meaning and that (successful) communication can be said to have occurred only when the listener manages to interpret these intentions and beliefs.

It may be worth pausing for a moment to consider what the role of linguistic comprehension is in real communicative situations. The purpose of comprehension is for one to be able to do something with the comprehended message (for example, to provide an appropriate answer; to make a relevant next contribution in conversation; to further one's knowledge; to amuse oneself and others). If one comprehends linguistically alone, then one cannot do anything with the message, since it does not connect with anything. We may further ask whether only linguistic comprehension is being tested in situations where a child needs to act on the comprehended message. Consider a comprehension test where a child is to choose a picture (from a set of pictures) which best demonstrates a given sentence. It would seem that to be able to choose a picture one needs more than linguistic comprehension. One needs to be able to put the sentence into an appropriate context – that is, to comprehend it pragmatically. If a child had particular difficulty with pragmatic comprehension, it would then follow that s/he could have difficulty with the above kind of comprehension tests and that this difficulty would not necessarily reflect linguistic comprehension difficulty. Tests of linguistic skills aim to eliminate the need to process contextual information, but it may not be possible to eliminate such processing completely given the nature of language comprehension. Somewhat paradoxically, however, children with pragmatic impairments may sometimes perform better under test conditions than one would expect given their performance in conversational settings, because of the exclusion of as many contextual variables as possible from linguistic tests.

Language as part of communication is characterized by uncertainty which the listener tries to minimize or eradicate when comprehending an expression. There are many sources of indeterminacy. Word meanings are frequently inherently ambiguous (I had to *put down* the cat). Novel uses of words, including creative idioms and non-literal expressions, can create uncertainty, as can syntactic ambiguity ('She approached the man with an axe'). As we saw above, pragmatic or discourse indeterminacy can stem from a variety of sources including speaker intention (Is s/he boasting or belittling?), implied meanings (Does saying X imply Y in this instance?) and indeterminate reference (Whom does 'he' refer to?). It seems remarkable that most indeterminacy goes unnoticed in successful everyday communication. It becomes resolved with reference to context (linguistic, discourse or physical) and/or the participants' world knowledge, including knowledge of one another. As speakers and listeners, we appear to be 'programmed' to focus on certain aspects of the message and context. It has been suggested that people tend to focus on what is relevant with regard to the ongoing discourse and what is most salient in the context (see also Chapter 7).

Inferencing and pragmatic comprehension

Making connections between pieces of information is important for the pragmatic comprehension of language expressions. The technical, cognitive psychology-based term for making connections is 'inferencing'. Inferencing refers to working on different sets of knowledge with a view to coming up with an outcome. In comprehension of language, inferencing adds information from memory to the current linguistic input to come up with a full or inferred interpretation. Two different types of inferencing processes are usually identified: deductive and inductive inferences.

In deduction, fixed rules are applied to information in order to arrive at an outcome. As such, deductive inferences are inflexible and not uncertain. Given a certain premise, the outcome simply follows from that, because of rules of logic.

(1) If the eggs are incubated for 20 days, they will hatch.
(2) The eggs are incubated for 20 days.
Outcome: The eggs will hatch.

Given the state of affairs in (1) and (2), *the only possible outcome* is the one stated. One does not need to think any further, but simply apply a rule of logic.

Inductive inferences, however, are quite different in that they do not neatly follow from a given premise by a simple application of rules. They are just *plausible outcomes* given the available information. In a way, making inductive inferences rests on guessing what might happen or what the situation might turn out to be.

(1) Bears like eating honey.
(2) There is a bear eating something in that tree.
A possible outcome: The bear in the tree is eating honey.

This outcome does not necessarily follow from (1) and (2) since it is possible, for instance, that the bear is not eating honey at that time. There are other possible scenarios which would then produce different possible outcomes. The point is that, depending on how the world is and how we, as interpreters, perceive it at a given point in time, this gives rise to different ways of making sense of the world and the incoming input. This gives rise to different inductive inferences. In this way an inductive inference does not follow automatically by application of rules of logic, but it is only a plausible conclusion that the comprehender works out on the basis of available evidence.

Pragmatic comprehension, going beyond the language expression itself, can be said to involve both deductive and inductive inferencing. We will explain this further in Chapter 7. Meanwhile, it suffices to note that when trying to work out what an expression means, we are involved in putting together information to produce an uncertain meaning. The meaning is uncertain because the context that one has built for interpretation may not be an appropriate one and/or can change as a consequence of new incoming information.

EXERCISE 6.2

The concepts of deductive and inductive inferencing are relevant to thinking about pragmatic impairment in children. Here are some statements about inferencing and pragmatic impairment and we would ask you to say whether the statements are likely to be *true* or *false* and *why*.

(1) Some children may find it easier to engage in deductive inferencing than inductive inferencing.
(2) If a child has problems with inferencing then pragmatic comprehension difficulties will ensue.

(3) Children who have problems with pragmatic comprehension would not benefit from therapy which builds on their ability to make plausible guesses on the basis of given input.

(4) What may seem like problems with inferencing may in fact reflect lack of world knowledge or even lack of confidence.

Comment 6.2

(1) This is likely to be true, since deductive inferencing is more fixed and rule-governed than inductive inferencing. For some children it is likely to be easier to work out outcomes when no uncertainty is involved in the process. Inductive inferencing is uncertain, resulting only in possible outcomes, which can change if new information becomes available and, as a consequence, more cognitive 'flexibility' is required to deal with such uncertainty. Some children may be drawn towards scientific subjects in school where logical inference is all-important.

(2) This is likely to be true, since to be able to comprehend the pragmatic (intended) meaning of an utterance one needs to engage in the uncertain process of working out what the meaning of the utterance might be on the basis of any available evidence. Inferencing enables the listener to go beyond what has been explicitly stated in the language expression, to the sphere of implied meaning.

(3) This is likely to be false, since pragmatic comprehension rests on 'guessing' the intended meaning of the utterance on the basis of language input and any other available evidence. Children with pragmatic comprehension difficulties may have a particular problem with such 'guessing' and would therefore make only limited gains if pressed to learn more about logical connections.

(4) This is true, since one's knowledge of the world forms the basis for inferencing. We make connections on the basis of what we know and the input that we receive. So, what may seem on the surface to be a problem of making connections (inferencing) may in fact reflect lack of world knowledge. Similarly, because comprehending pragmatically is a rather uncertain process, a child may lack confidence in engaging fully in such an activity, particularly if his/her self-esteem happens to be low.

* * * * * *

It is clear from the discussion so far that comprehension is heavily embedded in cognition. Long- and short-term memory, reasoning skills, knowledge and meta-representation, integration and thinking are central to the whole process, from the construction of linguistic meaning to the arrival at the full (pragmatic) interpretation. A grasp of time and space concepts is also intrinsically linked to pragmatic comprehension. It is important to appreciate that comprehension problems may have an underlying cognitive explanation (see further Chapter 7).

Comprehension of questions

Children's daily communications with others, particularly in the school context, involve to a large extent the answering of questions. Questions can be seen to place differing pragmatic demands on a child. They can be said to carry varying inferential loads. What this means is that in order to answer a question one may need to do different amounts of piecing together of information (inferencing) to arrive at an answer. It may be easier to piece together information that is explicitly stated, or given, than to deal with information that has to be inferred beyond what is given. Imagine that the following short story and the two questions about it were presented to a young child. Would you think that one of the questions would be easier to answer than the other, and if so why?

> Mary has a playhouse in the garden. One day there was a great storm and it rained very heavily. Nobody had thought about the leaky roof. The floor was flooded.

Questions:
- (A) Where is Mary's playhouse? (in the garden)
- (B) Why was the floor flooded? (because of the leaky roof the rain from the storm could get inside the playhouse)

Assuming that the child has no attention or memory problems, the first question is likely to be easier to answer than the second. This is because the answer to the first question is explicitly stated in the story and the child does not need to inference or imagine beyond what is said to him/her. With regard to the second question, however, the child needs to go beyond the story itself by making connections on the basis of his/her world knowledge. We can say that the first question involves less inferencing than the second question. We can say that the inferential load of the second question is greater than that of the first question. The first type of question can be called a descriptive question in that the answer is found in the story description. The second type of question can be called an inferential question in that the answer is inferred beyond explicit description. This distinction between different types of question can be, and has been, used in studying children's pragmatic difficulties and can provide a helpful way forward for assessing (children's) pragmatic comprehension problems (Bishop and Adams, 1992; Leinonen and Letts, 1997b).

Exercise 6.3

Here is another short story and a set of questions associated with it. Your task is to decide which questions are descriptive and which are inferential.

> Mary went to buy some bread. She couldn't find her money. She emptied her pockets on the counter. She searched around the shop. She thought that she would have to go home without the bread. 'Never mind' said the shopkeeper 'you can pay next time.'

(1) What did Mary go to buy?
(2) Why did she empty her pockets on the counter?
(3) Had the money dropped on to the floor?
(4) Who said 'Never mind, you can pay next time'?
(5) Did Mary go home with or without the bread?

Comment 6.3

(1) This question can be said to be a descriptive question in that the answer is explicitly stated in the story ('Mary went to buy some bread').
(2) This can be said to be an inferential question in that the answer needs to be inferred beyond the story. The following kind of reasoning would have to take place. Mary emptied her pockets on the counter to look for her money as money can be carried in a pocket.
(3) This can be said to be an inferential question. To find the answer that the money had most likely not dropped on to the floor one would need to go through the following kind of reasoning: 'Mary searched around the shop' can mean that she looked on the floor too. She must have not found the money on the floor as she thought that she could not buy any bread and would need to go home without it. Had she found the money on the floor she would not have thought the above. So, the money had not dropped on to the floor.
(4) This can be said to be a descriptive question as the answer is explicitly stated in the story ('the shopkeeper said').
(5) This can be said to be an inferential question. To find the answer one needs to interpret the shopkeeper's words to mean 'You can take the bread now and pay for it next time you visit the shop as you don't have money with you now'. In other words, one needs to infer beyond what is explicitly stated.

What this exercise highlights is that questions that we ask children vary in terms of the work that they have to do to go beyond what is verbally given to them. We can say that the processing demands associated with questions vary. In other words, some questions seem to require more processing than others and in this way some questions can be said to be more difficult or complex. It is interesting to note, however, that the linguistic form of the question does not seem to be connected with the processing demands that it places on the child. It is customarily thought that 'why' questions are the hardest to answer, but, as we see in this exercise, the third question of the form 'Had the money dropped on to the floor?' is in fact more complicated to answer. Some careful thought could usefully be given to the types of question that we ask children: to the processing load that they carry and how the questions affect children's ability to provide acceptable answers. We shall return to these issues later in this chapter (see also Chapter 7).

EXERCISE 6.4

Our account of the comprehension process so far suggests what can go wrong with this process and what could usefully be kept in mind when looking into children's comprehension problems. Here is a checklist of the main points made so far. Your task is to consider whether the statements are likely to be *true* or *false*.

(1) Comprehension is a certain process.
(2) Pragmatic comprehension is based on the ability to make plausible inferences (or guesses) on the basis of language input and world knowledge.
(3) Linguistic comprehension rests on semantic and syntactic knowledge.
(4) Comprehension involves only linguistic comprehension.
(5) It may be difficult to test linguistic comprehension with children who have pragmatic comprehension problems.
(6) Pragmatic comprehension deficits may stem from lack of world knowledge.

Comment 6.4

(1) This is false, since the linguistic expression is not a reliable indicator of what the expression means, and, when working out the intended meaning, there are many possible interpretations. Hence comprehension is an uncertain process.
(2) This is true since to comprehend beyond what is linguistically stated (that is, pragmatically) one needs to put linguistic and other knowl-

edge together (that is, to inference) in order to arrive at the intended meaning.

(3) This is true given the way we have defined linguistic comprehension, but see also Chapter 7 where we refer to the difficulty involved in determining where the boundaries of semantic and pragmatic comprehension are.

(4) This is false as in real communicative situations one would always need to infer beyond what is linguistically expressed.

(5) This is likely to be true when considering tests where one needs to put the tested sentence into a context in order to understand it. However, the testing of comprehension of single words may involve only linguistic processing. More thought needs to be given to these important issues.

(6) This is true in the sense that if one does not have adequate world/experiential knowledge to draw on one cannot come up with the inferences needed for interpretation.

Developmental notes

As we have seen so far, comprehension of language in real communicative contexts is a complex process. To develop an adult capacity to comprehend language and connected discourse is a long process that continues well into adolescence. In some ways, becoming a more competent comprehender can be thought of as being a lifelong quest that is tied to continuing acquisition of world knowledge and experience. The linguistic and cognitive skills that form the basis for comprehension are, however, mastered in childhood and adolescence. Our purpose here is not to provide a comprehensive review of literature on normal acquisition of language comprehension, but simply to note some key points about this process.

The following quote from Milosky (1992) summarizes what seems central to the development of comprehension skills:

> ... [I] consider the developmental process as one of *increasingly sophisticated uses of context*. Development will be characterised in terms of *increasing fluidity or lack of rigidity in using context* and by changes in *the amount and kinds of knowledge* children acquire and use for *dealing with the basic indeterminacy in language* (Milosky, 1992:21) (emphasis added).

EXERCISE 6.5

We have emphasized what we consider key phrases in the above quotation. On the basis of this, consider the following questions:

(1) What is the context like in which children first begin to comprehend language?

(2) What does using context mean in the early development of comprehension?

(3) How can the use of context in comprehension become more sophisticated?

(4) Why is the increase in knowledge and experience relevant to the development of comprehension?

(5) Why do children need to become better at dealing with indeterminacy in language?

Comment 6.5

(1) Children begin their development by being bound to familiar and concrete contexts.

(2) In order to comprehend the meaning of what is said to them, children combine information from situation, environment and the non-verbal behaviours of the partner even before they can utilize the verbal input they receive. Intonation and stress patterns in the input are also thought to be important for early interpretation.

(3) From a very early age children are able to combine items of information to work out meanings (to inference). This ability becomes more sophisticated with children's increasing ability to inference on the basis of more subtle clues and beyond the immediate context. Both the amount of information available and the ability to combine one type of information with another increases with age.

(4) Acquisition of world knowledge and experience add to more sophisticated inferencing. In terms of language comprehension, inferencing is reflected in the ability to go beyond the linguistic message to the understanding of inferred and non-literal meanings. Comprehension of less contextually obvious intended meanings (for example, irony, lying, boasting) does not become possible until the school years.

(5) Language is full of uncertainty and ambiguity, and comprehension itself is an uncertain process. As children develop, they need to become more aware of this and they need to become better at dealing with such indeterminacy in order to comprehend language as it was intended to be comprehended. They need also to become aware that because of this uncertainty, communicative partners commonly check on one another's meaning and comprehension, 'negotiating' the joint creation of meaning.

Children's ability to answer questions is connected with their increasing competence in understanding implied meanings. Children's communication with adults, particularly in the school context, is sometimes focused around question–answer situations. Although various patterns can be found in children's comprehension of the grammatical form of question (for example, labelling questions or yes/no questions are easier to answer than open-ended questions), it has been emphasized in the literature that the pragmatic or functional requirements of questions have a strong bearing on the appropriacy of children's answers. The presence or absence of objects that are talked about or the immediacy of referential sources are part of the pragmatic environment that affects children's ability to provide adequate answers. When a child can answer a question of a particular grammatical form in one context but not in another we are alerted to the fact that influences other than linguistic ones are likely to be affecting the child's comprehension. Parnell and Amerman (1983) maintain that when considering children's mastery of question understanding, it is important to consider not only the structural nature of questions but also the child's:

(A) understanding of the purpose of the question
(B) understanding of the semantics of the proposition
(C) understanding of his/her own role as the recipient of the question
(D) willingness to fulfil the respondent role
(E) world knowledge to draw on.

Research has begun to address the kinds of variables that bear on children's understanding of questions. Pragmatic demands of questions relate partly to the processing demands that they place on the child, partly to the availability of the information needed in order to answer the question, and partly to the child's ability to utilize this information in providing the answer to the question (see further Chapter 7).

Studies of poor comprehenders

Children's comprehension skills can vary considerably. Children with expressive language difficulties may demonstrate subtle comprehension deficits, particularly with regard to more complex grammatical patterns (Bishop, 1979, 1982). The work of Conti-Ramsden, Crutchley and Botting (1997) has shown how comprehension and expressive difficulties can co-occur in specifically language-disordered children. An early study by Bishop (1982) showed that children with Landau-Kleffner syndrome, a condition that is characterized by regression of early normal language development affecting particularly receptive skills, exhibit idiosyncratic and deviant patterns of language comprehension which indicate difficulties with handling the hierarchical structure of language. Bishop's study further showed that the comprehension difficulties manifested in auditory, written and signed modalities, thus suggesting some common core difficulty that may be independent of language modality.

Work, particularly in psychology, has looked into the development of inferential skills in comprehension of language and discourse. Studies by Oakhill and colleagues (Oakhill, 1984; Oakhill and Yuill, 1986; Oakhill, Yuill and Parkin, 1986) have suggested the following of 7–8-year-old, less skilled comprehenders (these were children with poor 'normal' ability rather than children with any identifiable developmental difficulty):

(1) Poor comprehenders may find it difficult to keep track of pronoun (or anaphoric) links in discourse. The children in the Oakhill studies were not helped by clear gender clues (for example, 'Peter lent 10 pence to *Liz*, because *she* was very poor' versus 'Peter lent 10 pence to *Max*, because *he* was very poor'). Gender clues are generally helpful in pronoun resolution, thus suggesting that some unusual comprehension strategies may have been in play.
(2) Poor working memory and lack of world knowledge did not seem to contribute to the children's poor comprehension skills, but rather it was concluded that these particular poor comprehenders had difficulty with the accessing of inferential or implied meanings in the input texts.

Oakhill (1984) suggests that remedial procedures could usefully focus on the construction of meaning from text and on bringing knowledge from outside the text into this process. It may also be useful to teach strategies for organizing and retrieving information.

It is now well attested that language-disordered children may have cognitively based difficulties, particularly with regard to symbolic play, conceptual development, mental rotation, anticipatory imagery and processing capacity and skills, including inference construction (see Johnston and Smith, 1989; Bishop, 1991; Johnston, Smith and Box, 1997). Cognitive deficits are likely to affect pragmatic comprehension, given the nature of pragmatic comprehension. Weismer (1985) found that a group of language-disordered children scored significantly lower on spatial and causal inferences associated with both verbally and pictorially presented stories than groups of language and cognitive-matched normally functioning children. Their performance was, however, more similar to the vocabulary comprehension matched children than the cognitively matched children. These findings point to a cognitively based deficit which hinders the children's ability to piece together information and 'read between the lines' in order to arrive at a full understanding of a message. Crais and Chapman (1987) arrived at a similar conclusion in their study of story recall and inferencing skills of older (9–10-year-old) language-disordered children. Their study pointed to further difficulties with 'on-the-spot' inferencing in story recall, which in turn may be connected with difficulties of general 'on-line' processing.

Comprehension difficulties and pragmatic impairment

It is clear from theoretical perspectives and research on language-disordered children that children with pragmatic difficulties are highly likely to exhibit various types of comprehension deficit. There has been only minimal targeted research on this to date (Bishop and Adams, 1992; Vance and Wells, 1994; Leinonen and Letts, 1997b; Kerbel and Grunwell, 1998a and b; see Bishop, 1997 for a review of relevant research), but in clinical reports and observations frequent reference is found to difficulties that (can) reflect poor pragmatic comprehension. These include:

- expression may be superior to comprehension
- there may be problems in 'using context in comprehension'
- there may be difficulty with the comprehension of non-literal messages (for example, idiom comprehension)
- answering (some) questions may cause difficulty
- problems talking about topics which are divorced from the here and now may exist
- there may be difficulty maintaining topics in discourse
- the understanding of cause–effect and temporal–causal relationships may be poor
- problems with verbal reasoning may exist
- there may be a difficulty in drawing inferences about actions
- there may be some inflexibility in drawing inferences
- the processing of whole utterances or selecting relevant parts may present difficulty
- there may be a tendency to give too much or too little information

(for example, Prutting and Kirchner, 1983; Rapin and Allen, 1983, 1987; McTear, 1985a; Conti-Ramsden and Gunn, 1986; Jones, Smedley and Jennings, 1986; Culloden, Hyde-Wright and Shipman, 1986; Bishop and Rosenbloom, 1987; Adams and Bishop, 1989; Bishop and Adams, 1989; Hyde-Wright and Cray, 1991; Leinonen and Letts, 1997b; Kerbel and Grunwell, 1998a and b; Leinonen and Kerbel, 1999).

Potential comprehension deficits in pragmatic impairment have been further acknowledged in clinical pragmatic profiles, which include categories for focusing on comprehension difficulties. The 'Pragmatics/ Discourse Coding System' of Letts and Reid (1994), for instance, includes such categories as 'complete topic shift' (a child ignores an adult initiation by producing an irrelevant contribution), 'problem with the scope of initiation' (a child produces a response that is too general or specific) and 'discourse implications not understood' (a child fails to understand what is required by a particular situation). These and similar categories of other pragmatics profiles may be used to profile pragmatic comprehension deficits. What are needed now are more specific investigations of pragmatically impaired children's comprehension abilities, which will then lead to more focused clinical assessment tools.

Craig and Evans (1993) make the important point that SLI children's pragmatic and discourse skills may vary relative to their language comprehension abilities. They found that SLI children with expressive and receptive deficits performed significantly worse on certain measures of turn-taking and cohesion than children with primarily expressive deficits. These differences could not be explained by a reduced linguistic repertoire, but rather the answer seemed to lie more solidly in the children's comprehension difficulties. One way forward when considering SLI (and pragmatically impaired) children's comprehension abilities is to focus on their pragmatic and discourse behaviours with the view to trying to explain how the behaviours come about (see Chapter 7; also Leinonen and Kerbel, 1999).

Bishop and Adams (1992) looked at the comprehension of literal and inferential meaning by 61 SLI and pragmatically impaired (PI) children (age range 8–12 years). The children were questioned about stories that were presented either verbally or pictorially. Half the questions were 'descriptive' in the sense that the answer was mentioned in the story or was shown explicitly in the pictures. The other half required the children to go beyond the mentioned or presented, that is to make inferences beyond the input. Overall, both the SLI and the PI children performed significantly worse than control children on these story comprehension tasks, yet the question type ('descriptive' versus 'inferential') or mode of presentation (verbal or pictorial) did not differentiate between the groups. There was, however, a non-significant trend for the PI group to perform more poorly than the SLI children with inferential questions. Bishop and Adams note that on the basis of clinical observations it would have been expected that inferential comprehension would have been problematic for the PI children. They consider reasons such as the possible heterogeneity of the PI population as a potential explanation for the non-significant result in the study.

Another study that has focused specifically on PI children's pragmatic comprehension skills is that of Vance and Wells (1994). Eighteen normal and 18 SLI children, some with the clinical picture of PI, were given non-literal expressions to comprehend, on the basis of which they were to choose a picture (out of three options) that best described the depicted situation. The control children were 6–7-year-olds and the SLI children's ages ranged from 7;10 to 13;1. The children were matched on receptive language scores. No significant differences were found in the children's ability to understand the expressions. The error type (literal or irrelevant picture choice) did not differentiate between the groups either. All children were also able to interpret a sentence with a live metaphor (one which they could not have learned as a whole item), thus suggesting that they all had an ability to use a metaphoric strategy.

These findings suggest that the development of comprehension of non-literal meaning was not delayed or disordered in these particular SLI and PI children and consequently that this may not be a valid diagnostic feature of PI. This interpretation did not, however, accord with clinical observations where, using a checklist approach, therapists and teachers would describe the PI children as having 'a poor "ability to use context to deduce meaning"' (Vance and Wells 1994: 38). Various explanations are offered for this apparent discrepancy. One suggested reason is that at least some of the expressions used by Vance and Wells (for example, 'raining cats and dogs', 'be in the dog house', 'bull in a china shop') are likely to be learned as whole lexical units, thus calling for more linguistic than pragmatic comprehension. A further point made by Vance and Wells, although perhaps insufficiently stressed, is that, whereas the PI children did seem able to understand non-literal meaning when they had been alerted to the need to do so, they did not seem to realize when it was necessary to do so in real situations. Given all this, it seems to us that the overall conclusion which states that:

> on the evidence of research carried out to date, it seems quite possible that clinicians and researchers have got hold of the wrong end of the stick in assuming that there are underlying cognitive and semantic deficits that give rise to the communication problems of children with so-called semantic-pragmatic disorder (Vance and Wells, 1994: 43)

is unwarranted at the present.

The work of Kerbel and Grunwell (1998a) showed how research methodology can have an effect on how children perform on an idiom comprehension task. Their study of 26 pragmatically impaired children (aged between 6 and 11 years) indicated that when the children had to give a verbal definition of an idiom they performed more poorly as compared with when they acted out the same idiom on a play task. This same pattern was evidenced in two groups of normally functioning children and a group of language-disordered children without semantic/pragmatic difficulties. Interestingly, the definition task proved particularly difficult for the language impaired children (the ones without semantic/pragmatic deficits) so that a significant difference that was found between this and the pragmatically impaired group on the play task disappeared altogether. This may not be too unexpected since by definition the language impaired children had difficulty with expressive language, and hence providing verbal definitions is likely to be problematic. What is very interesting, however, is that the pragmatically impaired group differed from the language impaired group in this, which then indicates that this group was indeed pragmatically impaired rather than 'language impaired' and that clinical judgement had been able to put the children into the groups appropriately. The finding that all the children had more difficulty with providing definitions than with acting out the idioms confirms work that shows that there is a discrepancy between what a child knows and what a child is able to (verbally) demonstrate that s/he knows.

In a companion study, using the same children and the same play-based methodology as before, Kerbel and Grunwell (1998b) found that the pragmatically impaired children were significantly worse at idiom interpretation than the other three groups. The children's inappropriate interpretations tended to fall into the category of 'fuzzy actions' rather than 'literal interpretation'. Kerbel and Grunwell exemplify these two categories as follows. One of the idioms to be interpreted is in the sentence: 'Suddenly the bike rider stopped *on the spot.*' A literal interpretation would be recorded if a child stopped the bike rider on a green dot on the play set. A fuzzy interpretation would be evidenced if a child moved the already stationary bike rider to another location. Kerbel and Grunwell maintain that the difficulty pragmatically impaired children had with idiom comprehension, as evidenced by fuzzy rather than literal interpretations, indicates awareness that a literal interpretation is not appropriate. The fuzzy interpretations may further indicate that there is difficulty with retrieval of known idioms from memory and/or with the choosing of the most appropriate meaning when there are a number of possibilities. Despite their difficulties, the pragmatically impaired group had more appropriate interpretations than inappropriate ones. This may reflect the relative simplicity, from the pragmatics perspective, of the comprehension task used. The meanings of the idioms were relatively constrained in the given contexts in that the only other plausible interpretation was a literal one in that context. In 'real' communicative contexts pragmatic meanings are more fluid and subject to greater contextual variation.

Leinonen and Letts' (1997b) case study of a pragmatically impaired child, Sarah (10 years old), shows clearly how the pragmatic nature of the input question can have an effect on a child's ability to provide an appropriate answer. Sarah had particular difficulty with questions that required her to go beyond visually presented information or beyond verbally stated information. On one set of tasks she was to answer questions on the basis of composite pictures: for some of the questions, the answer was obvious from the picture (descriptive questions) and for others information needed to be inferred beyond the picture (for example, by imagining what had happened before and what is likely to happen next). Sarah's performance was much poorer on the inferential questions than on the descriptive questions and much poorer than the performance of 6- and 8-year-old normally functioning control children. Although the control children also found the inferential questions more difficult than the descriptive questions, this difficulty was not as pronounced as Sarah's. The trend was also apparent in a set of tasks that required the children to answer questions on the basis of verbally told stories. The study led Leinonen and Letts to suggest that pragmatically impaired children may have difficulty going beyond explicitly presented information. This would manifest as pragmatic production and comprehension problems. In cognitive terms, this may indicate difficulty with the process of inferencing.

In a discussion paper Leinonen and Kerbel (1999) explore how pragmatic comprehension difficulties can be examined from the relevance theory perspective (Sperber and Wilson, 1995). By focusing on data they show how the theory enables one to break down the comprehension process into component parts and how this enables an informed and illuminating exploration of children's comprehension difficulties. The paper shows how a great deal remains to be investigated and proposes some ways forward within the theory of relevance. This work is described in more detail in Chapter 7.

Clinical data

We will now aim to illustrate many of the points made in this chapter by considering data from two children with pragmatic difficulties.

EXERCISE 6.6

Read the following short data sample from Simon (10 years old), who has pragmatic difficulties (see also Chapters 4 and 5). Simon (S) is interacting with two adults. A1 is his speech and language therapist (one of the authors) and A2 is a technician who is videoing the session. Simon has an open story book on his lap (it has pictures and text) and is asked by A1 to tell the story to A2, who does not know the story. A1 and Simon have shared the story on previous occasions.

In the story, a boy is having a dream about a gorilla and himself and various adventures that they get into. The boy and the gorilla made a mess in the story, which they then attempted to clear up. The boy's father was cross with them and the boy promised to be good. On the page that is open at this point, the boy is asleep in his bed with a 'dream-bubble' above his head. There is a picture of a gorilla in the bubble.

In the transcript, square brackets designate overlapping utterances and Simon's inappropriate contributions (*) are identified by letters for ease of reference. Ignore, for the moment, the numbers after some of the adults' utterances. We have discussed in Chapter 1 the difficulties involved in making (in)appropriacy judgements. For the purposes of this exercise, Simon's answer is deemed inappropriate if it does not provide the answer required by the question. There is, of course, the important point of whether the adults' questions are appropriate to Simon's level of functioning. We shall consider this in Exercise 6.7 below. The judgements of inappropriacy with regard to these data are based on a study (Leinonen and Smith, 1994) in which we had asked more than 50 people to identify instances of inappropriacy in this sample. In this way we feel more comfortable that the judgements should have at least some reality. It is important to note, however, that none of the people making the judgements were speech-language therapists, but they were people of varying professional backgrounds and students of education and linguistics.

S: He's in bed and he's a, and he sees a gorilla.
A1: Where does he see the gorilla?
S: In bed.(*) A
A1: In bed. Yes, but is it in his dreams, or is the gorilla on the ceiling, or, umm, is the gorilla sitting on the bed? (1)
S: Yes (*) B
A1: Which one?
S: The boy's.(*) C
A1: The boy's ...{rising intonation}
S: Bed
A1: Bed. Mmm. Simon, do you think they are good now [now or are they being more naughty than ever?]
S: [Yes] Yes.(*) D
A1: Which do you think? (2)
S: The gorilla.(*) E
A1: Listen. Are they going to be good or are they going to be naughty?
S: Naughty.
A1: Why? (3)
S: Because it's made a mess.(*) F

A1: Aah. That's what he was. He was naughty wasn't he.
A2: But what do you think they will be tomorrow? (4)
S: Clearing all the mess.(*) G
A1: You think they'll clear all the mess.
S: Yes.

To understand this story and, therefore, to be able to retell it and to answer the questions posed by the adults, Simon needs to have understood that the events were part of a dream (that is, imaginary) and that certain things happen in the story because of other events.

On the basis of the short data sample, consider:

(1) Whether you agree with our judgement that there is something communicatively peculiar in this sample and that Simon's contributions marked by (*) are inappropriate in the sense of not providing the answer required by the adult question.
(2) Whether this inappropriacy could reflect pragmatic comprehension difficulty and if so, state why.
(3) What kinds of demands the adult questions, which are followed by Simon's inappropriate answers, place on him? What do they require him to be able to do in order to be able to answer the questions?

Comment 6.6

In Chapter 1 we considered problems with inappropriacy judgements. You may not agree with our decisions here, but, for the sake of this exercise, you will need to consider our explanations for them.

(1) and (2). We consider the marked utterances inappropriate for the following reasons:

(A) The question asks Simon to refer to the boy having a dream (that is, the boy sees the gorilla in his dreams). Simon interprets the question very concretely, as depicted in the picture, in which the boy is lying in bed asleep. This could be considered a pragmatic problem in that the language expression is interpreted without taking the context into account (that is, the picture is not understood).

(B) and (D) Simon is answering questions of alternatives as a yes–no question. It may be that Simon is adopting a strategy of providing 'yes' as an answer whenever he has difficulty understanding a question. This could be indicative of a pragmatic comprehension problem which the 'yes' strategy is reflecting.

(C) and (E) Simon does not seem to understand that the questions 'which one' or 'which one do you think' ask him to make a choice between the alternatives provided in the adult's previous question. He interprets the first of these questions (in C) in relation to his previous idea that the boy is in his bed when he sees the gorilla. He interprets the second question (in E) as requiring him to specify who is being good or naughty. These kinds of problems could be considered pragmatic problems since they show that Simon has difficulty utilizing the previous discourse in making sense of the adult questions. These two questions cannot be interpreted without appropriate recourse to previous discourse.

(F) There are two problems in Simon's answer here and both can be said to be pragmatic in nature. First, it is not clear what the pronoun 'it' refers to. Pronouns are 'empty' words that gain their meaning from context. Second, the answer does not tell us why the gorilla and the boy are going to be naughty, but rather it attempts to say why they could be considered to have been naughty (that is, because they made a mess).

(G) The inappropriacy in this answer is very similar to the inappropriacy in many of the other utterances in that Simon is again answering the adult question in isolation from the previous discourse and in a very concrete manner. The question is still attempting to elicit an answer to the initial good/naughty question, but Simon interprets it as being quite separate. The adult question means 'Do you think that the boy and the gorilla are going to be good or naughty tomorrow?' but Simon had interpreted it to mean 'What do you think the boy and the gorilla will be doing tomorrow?', to which he answers 'Clearing all the mess'. This kind of a misinterpretation can again be described as reflecting problems with pragmatic comprehension (see further Chapter 7).

(3) The adult uses a variety of question forms (for example, which, why, given alternative questions) and Simon does not seem to have particular difficulty with any one type of question. Simon's difficulty with the given alternative questions is reflected in his tendency to provide a 'yes' answer before the question is completed. These questions require him to consider evidence, weigh it up and come up with a considered answer. The questions can be said to be inferential in nature. To be able to answer the questions he needs to understand the story and particularly why events occur. If one does not understand the story line, then the best one can do is to describe the story in fairly concrete terms, perhaps as depicted in associated pictures. Simon's answers indicate that this is what he is doing much of the time. Three of the adult (in C, E and G) questions also require Simon to understand that the question refers to previous discourse.

When in conversation with communicatively limited clients it is necessary for skilled clinicians to be able to do two things:

(1) To judge whether the client's utterances would or would not pass as acceptable outside the clinical situation.
(2) To interpret his or her utterances as generously as possible, at times when the client is not being assessed, making allowances for any difficulties and adapting to them in the way that most people do quite naturally when talking with a young child. As the child's communication improves other intervention strategies may become more appropriate.

These principles enable the clinician to have a realistic view of the client's needs and enable the client to experience conversational success, thereby gaining confidence, self-esteem, motivation and experience of how conversation works.

During the above interaction both adults attempt to converse with Simon as if he were able to function normally.

EXERCISE 6.7

Your task is now to consider why we have judged some of the adult utterances in the transcript to be inappropriate in that they would not serve the second purpose we describe above. That is to say, they are not maximally facilitative. The inappropriate utterances are numbered on the data transcript.

Comment 6.7

(1) Given that Simon probably felt that he had answered the question correctly and that the adult had failed to make clear exactly what she wanted to know, a more constructive reply would be possible, for example: 'Yes, the boy was in bed when he saw the gorilla'; 'Where was the gorilla?'
(2) Here the confusion deepens because Simon is not helped to see exactly what the question refers to. A reflection would probably be more validating here, for example: 'You think they will be naughty.'
(3) Again, it is not made clear to Simon that the question means 'why do you think what you have just said you think?' The question 'Why?' is dependent on context. It would help to carry the interaction forward if A1 supported Simon's statement, for example: 'Yes they seem to like being naughty'; or 'Yes. I think you're right.'

(4) To begin with 'but' introduces a doubt. Also the question is ambiguous. Simon assumes that it means 'what will they be doing?' not 'will they be naughty or good?' The only way that he can be sure that the second possible meaning is the intended one is by having a clear idea of the topic which is uppermost in the minds of his co-interactants. He might need help with this, for example: 'So we're thinking about whether they will be naughty or good'; 'I wonder what will happen tomorrow?'; or 'I wonder if tomorrow will be the day when they start to be good?'

EXERCISE 6.8

Sarah (10 years old) is performing a task with one of the authors (Leinonen and Letts, 1998b). She is shown a composite picture of a park and is asked questions about it. In the picture there are two men sitting on a bench, one eating lunch and the other reading a newspaper. The men are in work overalls. In front of the men there is a hole which has been recently dug, and there are a spade and digging tools around the hole. Next to the hole there is a tree lying on the ground. There are also two other trees freshly planted near the hole. There is a hut in the park and there is a man in the hut. Near the hut there is a fence to which a dog is tied by its lead. There are no leaves on the trees and there are some daffodils in bloom. The sky is grey.

Your first task is to read through this short data sample.

A: *Is there someone in the hut?* (1) (points to a hut/there is a man in it)
S: No.(*)
A: OK. *What are the two men doing on the bench?* (2)
S: Mmm sitting. That one's reading the paper and that one's gone to sleep.
A: Yeah. He looks a bit tired (laughs)
S: (laughs)
A: *What is this?* (3) (points to a bridge)
S: Mmm a bridge.
A: That's right. *Are dogs allowed to run free?* (4) (points to a dog that is tied to a fence by its lead)
S: No.
A: *Why is that?* (5)
S: Because he's got a collar.(*)
A: Yeah. That's right. *What season of the year is it?* (6)
S: I think it's spring.
A: Mmm *Why is that?* (7).
S: Mmm—It's a sunny day (points to blue sky; there is no sun)
A: Yeah. It's sunny, isn't it.
S: (laughs)
A: *What is this place?* (8)
S: Err–I think it's a garden.
A: Sorry. Can you say that again.

S: I think it's a garden.

A: You think it's a garden.

S: Yeah.

A: Yes. That's a good thing. *Are the men going to do any more work?* (9) (points to the two workmen on the bench)

S: No.(*)

A: OK. *Why is that?* (10)

S: Because they (an unintelligible/inaudible word) have the rest.(*)

A: They are having a rest.

S: Yeah.

A: *How many garden tools are there?* (11)

S: Mmm–three, four (points while counting)

A: Four yeah. You nearly forgot that one (laughs)

S: (laughs)

A: Mmm *What is the hole for?* (12) (the two workmen had been planting trees before their break. There are two trees planted in a row in two holes and there is a hole for a third tree which is lying on the ground next to the hole)

S: Mmm——(approx. 10 sec pause). I think it's for to put treasure in it (mumbled)(*)

A: To put a what?

S: A treasure.

A: Yeah could be. You could dig a hole for that, couldn't you. *How many trees are there in the picture?* (13)

S: One, two—six (points while counting)

A: Six trees. Yeah. Well done. You have done very well indeed. Shall we have a look at some other pictures?

S: Yeah (laughs)

You are now asked to

(1) Consider whether you agree with our judgements of which of Sarah's answers are inappropriate (those marked by *). Note again that an answer is deemed inappropriate if it does not provide the answer requested by the question. We are not concerned here with the important points of whether the questions themselves are fully appropriate for Sarah's level of functioning or whether it is appropriate to direct as many questions to children as the adults in this and the previous sample of Simon do. The inappropriacy judgements were made separately by two individuals (one of the authors and a research student) and disagreements were resolved by discussion. It is worth noting that it is much easier to decide what is inappropriate in relation to the present task than in relation to a more spontaneous conversation, since the pictures provide a clear point of reference for deciding the correctness of the answer.

(2) Decide which of the questions are descriptive (*desc*) or inferential (*infer*) (see Exercise 6.3 above).

(3) Consider whether Sarah seems to have problems with particular types

of questions (that is, *desc* or *infer*).

(4) Consider whether Sarah's comprehension problems could be considered pragmatic in nature.

Comment 6.8

(1 and 2) We considered the answers inappropriate for the following reasons and have decided on the nature of the questions as follows.

Question 1: The answer is blatantly wrong since there is a man in the hut. This is a *desc* question as the answer is visually given.

Question 5: The way to work out that dogs are not likely to be allowed to run free is not because the dog which is tied to the fence has a collar, but because it is likely that this particular dog is tied to the fence because dogs in general are not allowed to run free. This is an *infer* question as one needs to go beyond the picture to infer the answer.

Question 9: The picture indicates (as does the question itself) that the men have been working previously and are likely to be having a break now. The way their tools have been left around the hole, in addition to the two freshly planted trees plus the tree lying on the ground waiting to be planted, indicates that they are going to continue with work (planting) after their break. So, 'no' is not an appropriate answer. This is an *infer* question as one needs to put a great deal of information together from the picture and one's world knowledge to come up with the answer.

Question 10: It is not appropriate to infer that because the men are having a rest they are not going to do any more work. In fact, the very word 'rest' implies that more work is to be done. This is an *infer* question because one needs to go beyond the picture.

Question 12: As described in relation to question 9, the picture indicates that the hole is for planting the last tree. Sarah's answer is totally unconnected with this scenario and thus inappropriate. This is an *infer* question because one needs to put together information from various sources to come up with the answer.

(3) In this small data sample, Sarah has more difficulty with answering the inferential questions than the descriptive questions.

(4) To be able to comprehend pragmatically, one needs to be able to infer meaning beyond the immediate context, taking into account contextual features and one's world knowledge. Sarah's difficulty with inferential questions rather than descriptive questions would suggest a pragmatic type of problem, but more in-depth investigation would be needed to confirm this.

Linguistic interpretation

Form and function

For both Simon and Sarah, there was not a clear relationship between the linguistic form of the question and the appropriacy of the answer. Both children can be seen comprehending the same syntactic form in one context and yet not in another. This suggests that syntactic comprehension may not be a likely explanation of the observed difficulties but rather, that the children's comprehension problems reflect difficulty with functional (or inferential) demands of the input question. Both children do, however, have problems with 'why' questions. Normally developing children also have difficulty providing appropriate answers to these types of question, thus suggesting that these questions are somehow developmentally problematic. Similar problems have also been observed with SLI and pragmatically impaired children (for example, Conti-Ramsden and Gunn, 1986). 'Why' questions may be conceptually demanding in terms of reasoning and inferencing. Other data from Sarah suggest that the linguistic form of 'why' questions was not a problem for her since she answered 'why' questions appropriately on some occasions.

Inferential demands of questions

The analysis presented here would also suggest that the amount of information that was available for the children in the immediate context may have affected the children's ability to answer questions. It seemed for both children that the more the child was required to go beyond the concrete input (visual or verbal), the harder it became to produce an appropriate response. Simon, for instance, seemed to find it difficult to answer questions that required him to speculate or hypothesize about the likely (future) behaviour of the story characters (Are they going to be good or are they going to be naughty?). Similarly, Sarah's difficulties seemed to surface more clearly when she was required to move beyond the presented pictures. The important point to note here is that even though there seems to be a pattern whereby the inferential demands of the question relate to the appropriacy of the answer, this pattern does not confirm that the underlying problem is that of inferencing. It may well be associated with lack of world knowledge or confidence or with cognitively demanding concepts such as time and space.

Metacommunication

Communication about the communication process itself requires the ability to divorce oneself from the explicitly stated and move to a higher level of cognitive functioning (see further Smith and Leinonen, 1992). A child needs to realize that we can talk about the process that we are currently engaged in and that this is a way of organizing the path the communication is to take next. In the Simon sample there were some adult questions which had a metacommunicative function, and both children gave both appropriate and inappropriate answers. The samples are too small to find any patterns in them, but we can note that Simon had apparent difficulty appreciating that at one point the adults were trying to get him to choose between options given by their questions and were not asking him to focus on the content of the questions. One of the adults uses this kind of a question twice: 'Which one?' and 'Which do you think?' These questions mean 'Which one of the alternatives that I gave in the previous question do you want to choose?' In fact the questions mean, 'Choose one of the alternatives that I gave in my previous question.' In this way the adult questions focus on the communication process and the questions themselves rather than on the content of the story. These sorts of questions are likely to be particularly problematic for someone who has difficulty with metarepresentation.

Communication or compensatory strategies

One difficulty with relying on the surface behaviours as an indicator of possible comprehension problems is brought about by the fact that a child may be using communication or compensatory strategies to cope with a problem. Such strategies serve to minimize or even disguise the problem (see further Smith and Leinonen, 1992). It is commonly reported that linguistically and pragmatically impaired children tend to reply minimally (for example, 'yes', 'no', 'don't know', repetition of a word in the adult utterance) to adult questions/input and that these responses sometimes seem to serve the purpose of the child taking his/her turn without necessarily engaging in the conversation. With such responses it is difficult for the adult to know whether the child has actually responded appropriately, since the answer may by chance be a correct one. In the Simon sample, there were instances where the minimal answer was appropriate but when the child was asked for a justification for the answer, it became inappropriate.

Simon:
A: Listen. Are they going to be good or are they going to be naughty?
S: Naughty.
A: Why?
S: Because it's made a mess.(*)

For the more hypothetical and inferential questions, the child's true understanding can be revealed only by the justification given to a further 'why' question. To complicate matters, there is of course the possibility that the child knows the justification and has worked it out appropriately, but has problems with expressing this linguistically. Unresolved expressive difficulties can in this way lead to misjudged comprehension difficulties. The converse is true too, whereby comprehension difficulties may be masked by expressive linguistic problems.

One further effect of communication strategies on one's view of children's comprehension abilities concerns the control of topics in conversations. In spontaneous conversation, Sarah created the impression of a skilled and competent communicator and there did not seem to be any reason to believe that she had comprehension difficulties. This did not tally with reports of her class teacher and her speech-language therapist. A closer look at the successful conversations indicated that they were largely about topics chosen by Sarah and therefore it would often be impossible for the adult to know whether her contributions were appropriate, or even truthful. It was partly because of this difficulty that it seemed necessary to employ more controlled data collection procedures so that we were able to examine Sarah's comprehension difficulties in more detail.

Clinical interpretation

Clinicians are now well aware that, in assessing and treating comprehension, a distinction needs to be made between linguistic and pragmatic abilities. What is less well understood at present is the need to make other, more subtle, distinctions within the pragmatic category and to facilitate the acquisition and integration of all the skills and types of knowledge involved in situational comprehension. A familiar clinical experience is to find that clients perform differently in test situations and in spontaneous performance. This, too, has to be accommodated in working out how best to assess and remediate their problems. On the basis of material presented in this chapter it is possible at least to suggest some areas for consideration.

Comprehension as a basis for performance

We have suggested that it may be wise to keep in mind that in cases of inappropriate pragmatic behaviour there may be an underlying comprehension problem rather than an impairment in the ability to produce satisfactory pragmatic performance. It may well be that some type or degree of comprehension problem is preventing the client from weighing up what is needed in the way of a response. The data from Sarah and Simon show this possibility quite clearly.

Cognitive issues, world knowledge and experience

The ability to understand situations and utterances depends on the presence of several types of knowledge (linguistic, social and 'knowledge of the world') and on the ability to remember, integrate and spot the relevance of whatever knowledge we possess. Clearly, the inexperienced client whose environment has provided little access to the world or its inhabitants is at a disadvantage where pragmatic comprehension is concerned. The same may be true of the client whose early communication problems have reduced the amount of social learning that has taken place. Cognitive problems may prevent other individuals from acquiring knowledge even though opportunities are plentiful. A situation where a client cannot integrate or apply knowledge that is in place is more puzzling than the situation reflecting lack of knowledge or experience. Are the difficulties due to cognitive deficits or does the explanation lie in an emotional problem or lack of confidence? Will practice improve the client's performance? Only multidisciplinary approaches can provide satisfactory answers to these concerns.

A further cognitive impairment which can compromise pragmatic performance is slowness in processing what has just been said. This, especially when it is combined with slowness in designing and producing one's own utterance, can create the impression that totally inappropriate contributions are being offered. For instance, the reply intended to fit a previous question may be produced just as a new question has been uttered, or a reply may be given long after the questioner has lost interest. Simon had problems with the processing of incoming information at the speed that was needed in conversation. He demonstrated much better 'comprehension ability' when the pressure to process at 'normal comprehension speed' was removed.

Form, function and context

Clinical assessment and teaching routinely address clients' vocabulary and grammatical abilities; thus it would be unusual for a clinician to fail to realize that deficits in these areas were interfering with the ability to respond appropriately. What is perhaps more problematic is that knowledge of linguistic form does not guarantee its reliable use in comprehension any more than it does in production. Clinicians are familiar with the fact that words and grammatical constructions that clients can produce to order may never be used in real life. Similarly, the need to employ knowledge of a structure, an idiom or even a word in interpreting an utterance may not be as evident to clients as it is to clinicians. Another possibility is that the relevance of interpreting utterances in a particular way may not be obvious to clients for reasons of inexperience or disability. An example of failure to recognize the relevance of a particular way of interpreting would be one's initial difficulty in understanding a decontextualized sentence such as 'This particular witch was not much good at spelling' (casting spells).

It is thought (Vance and Wells, 1994; Leinonen, 1995) that one of the possibilities in cases of failure to use linguistic knowledge appropriately is that for some reason an individual may be unable, or unmotivated, to analyse the context of a remark efficiently or to identify correctly the topic that is being talked about. These skills seem sometimes to be affected by disability, but it is also possible that insufficient experience in interacting with facilitative partners accounts for a weakness of this kind. This notion raises the question of whether clinicians' own stimulus utterances to clients are always as appropriate as they could be (see Leinonen and Smith, 1994).

Clinicians need also to be aware that the interpretation of a speaker's intention (speech act) is necessary if the respondent is to design his or her own speech act appropriately in reply (for instance, to take a joke lightly or fit an answer to an indirect question). Training in this type of matching can help a client to fit more comfortably into social settings, for instance work or school, but before remediation can be offered a deficiency has first to be recognized.

The inferential load of questions to clients

In asking for an appropriate response to a question, one makes an assumption that the person responding will have understood more than the literal meaning of what has been said. Insufficient insight is currently available as to the *degree* of inferential load imposed by various types of questions and utterances, but it is essential to give some thought to the possibility that clients may find certain types easy or difficult to respond to for both linguistic and extralinguistic reasons. Inferences about what speakers mean by what they say are made on the basis of what we know about the speakers themselves, about various aspects of the context and about the way language can potentially be used. These are complex matters and it does not seem surprising that both normal communicators and those with communicative problems find difficulty with inferencing at times. Comprehension 'guesswork' seems to be easier for some individuals than for others and, given that the 'true' meaning of an utterance is often open to dispute (indeterminate), some training and encouragement for the ability to reason inductively can be very helpful. This is given through the formation of relationships and active involvement with facilitative communicative partners who are willing to tolerate ineptness and to provide plentiful demonstration and explanation in the early stages.

Metacommunication

It is not unusual for the utterances directed to clients to have a metacommunicative function. That is to say that the utterances are about the communication process itself. We saw in the data samples above how Simon had particular difficulty knowing that one of the adults was trying to get him to appreciate that she was asking forced alternative questions. To operate at a metarepresentational level of functioning is a highly demanding processing activity. Consider, for instance, the complex processing involved in answering 'No' to the seemingly simple question 'Do you understand?' It is not difficult to see how clients with processing difficulties may fail to comprehend metacommunicative input adequately. In this regard too, thought could usefully be given to the complexity of utterances addressed to pragmatically impaired clients.

Narratives

Narratives can be a fruitful medium for tuition in comprehending communicative intentions and implied meanings. The more time that is spent in constructing interesting narratives (not merely 'sequences') with clients and helping them to enjoy the stories told to them or reconstructed from cartoons or book illustrations, the more the possibility of narrative as a therapy tool reveals itself. Narrative has also proved helpful in enabling clients to learn how to keep track of the referents for pronouns within texts and encouraging them to expand their memory skills. There is also the possibility of persuading clients to take the risk, in pursuit of interest and amusement, of separating themselves from the security of 'the here and now'. This is a crucial step in gaining pragmatic flexibility and beginning to make use of imagination in interpreting other people's communicative needs and intents. Add to these advantages the considerable input of information, connected language, vocabulary and insight into other people's way of thinking, feeling and speaking that can be provided through the medium of stories, and their therapeutic potential is clear.

Communication strategies

Socially skilled clients sometimes adopt positive communication strategies (Smith and Leinonen, 1992). Although these can be valuable and should not be thoughtlessly discouraged, they can serve to mask comprehension difficulties which would be better revealed and treated. For instance, the understandable short-term wish to save face and keep an interaction going can motivate an individual to nod and smile at times when a more constructive strategy would be to ask for an explanation or to look puzzled. Clients who simulate comprehension can sometimes be labelled 'pragmatically skilled' when in fact they need help. Strategies can be, and are, taught to language impaired children. They can be encouraged to monitor input for things they do not understand, and make appropriate clarification requests. The question of how successful such techniques would be with pragmatically impaired children remains to be explored, but given the very nature of pragmatic impairments strategies taught to pragmatically impaired children may well need to be different from those used with language impaired children.

Developmental approach

Relatively little is known of the developmental progression of pragmatic comprehension or of the developmental relationship between linguistic comprehension and pragmatic performance. The development of speech act comprehension is reviewed in McTear and Conti-Ramsden (1992). The popular Dewart and Summers (1995) assessment and other pragmatic assessments such as those discussed by McTear and Conti-Ramsden and by Smith and Leinonen (1992) deal with pragmatic comprehension to some extent, but there have been few studies of the development of non-literal understanding. In these circumstances clinicians are thrown on their own resources if they wish to approach clients' difficulties from a developmental standpoint.

What is clear is that some level of inferencing plays a part in the human infant's early attempts to work out from personal and situational clues what other human beings are likely to mean by what they say. How else could it be done? If this notion is accepted, it follows that guesswork and experimentation need to be encouraged, preferably within stable supportive relationships, as a means of laying down the foundations for communicative and linguistic progress. Feeding, bathing, dressing, shopping, outings, and mutual involvement with pets, music, picture books and play provide the natural contexts for the acquisition, first of basic pragmatic knowledge and skill, and later of language and higher-level pragmatics. Clinicians are aware of the importance of concrete, non-verbal and situational support for the earliest stages of communicative development. They also emphasize the development of non-linguistic comprehension prior to speech and language.

What can be lost sight of is that pragmatic comprehension, through inferencing, also needs to be encouraged at an early stage. It seems possible that the later, more demanding inferencing which leads to the sophisticated interpretation of implied meanings requires this type of early experience to support it and may be inhibited by too great an emphasis on literal accuracy alone during the language acquisition period. Clearly, there is a danger that this might happen when clinicians set out to remediate language deficits. Thus it seems particularly desirable to give careful thought to the developmental primacy of communication and to then build linguistic skills on firm pragmatic foundations.

Summary

In this chapter we have discussed how comprehension involves the ability to manipulate both linguistic and contextual data (including world knowledge) and the ability to assess how those who interact with us process data. The linguistic expression itself is not a reliable indicator of what is meant by an utterance and the aim of comprehension is to come up with the intended, and only the intended, interpretation. When engaging in pragmatic comprehension we draw on a number of contextual resources. We need to be able to access and integrate data from various sources (memory, verbal and visual input) and we need to complete this process with sufficient speed in order to keep up with the demands of the communicative situation. The development of comprehension seems to involve an increasing ability to use context in discerning meaning, starting with the processing of information in the 'here and now' and moving on to the processing of hypothetical and imaginative data. Some studies of poor comprehenders have shown that the problems with the connectedness of ideas in discourse and the ability to 'read between the lines' may be linked more to inferencing abilities than to linguistic processing or memory skills. Poor comprehension can of course stem from a variety of sources, reflecting linguistic, cognitive (including memory, speed of processing, inferencing skills, the ability to manipulate the concepts of time and space and theory of mind abilities) and metarepresentational difficulties. Lack of or gaps in one's world knowledge, and difficulties associated with children's environments, can also be contributing factors. It is highly likely that many children who are currently described as having pragmatic impairments have comprehension difficulties that are pragmatic in nature. These difficulties would manifest in conversational inappropriacy and would most likely affect all forms of connected discourse. It seems a worthwhile way forward in our quest to understand more about the nature of children's pragmatic deficits to focus on pragmatic comprehension. We will discuss this further in the next chapter (Chapter 7).

Chapter 7: Pragmatic principles and relevance

Key words: pragmatic theory and explanation, the cooperative principle and Grice's maxims, implicatures, relevance theory, processing issues.

Aims

What is it that a theory of pragmatics attempts to do? As pragmatics is about contextual meaning, dealing with both its production and comprehension, thus a pragmatic theory aims to account for how it is that producers and receivers arrive at such meaning. Pragmatics rests on the assumption that communicative use of language involves meaning beyond the linguistic expression and its syntactic arrangement; that is, beyond what is explicitly stated. What is there beyond this? There are the intentions and beliefs of the speaker and hearer, their individual and shared knowledge and the context in which the utterance occurs (see Chapter 6 for an account of what are pragmatic aspects of meaning). All this gives rise to 'meaning beyond the words' and pragmatic theory tries to explain how. This chapter aims to explore the following:

> **Key questions:**
> What is the cooperative principle?
> What are implicatures?
> How does the cooperative principle try to account for implicatures?
> What is relevance theory?
> How does relevance theory try to account for pragmatic meaning?
> How could the knowledge of relevance theory help with our understanding of children's pragmatic difficulties?

The chapter aims to give a succinct account of Grice's (1975) cooperative principle and Sperber and Wilson's (1995) relevance theory. The primary focus of the chapter is on relevance theory, and Grice's theory will be examined only briefly as a background to the theory of relevance. Parts of this chapter will be based on the work of Leinonen and Kerbel (1999) on relevance theory and pragmatic impairment. The aim of this chapter is not to give a fully comprehensive overview of the two theories. For this the reader is referred to the original texts (and also Wilson and Sperber, 1981; Sperber and Wilson, 1987) and to such overviews as those given by Levinson (1983), Blakemore (1992) and Grundy (1995).

Background concepts and issues

Grice's cooperative principle

Grice (1975) started with the premise that people strive to behave in a rational and cooperative manner, rather than the opposite, when communicating with others. This being the case, according to Grice, speakers are assumed to operate within the cooperative principle and its four maxims and listeners also assume that speakers do this. As a consequence of these assumptions, contextual meanings arise and are interpreted.

The cooperative principle states that speakers aim to make their contribution in conversation which is relevant to the purpose and direction of the conversation. In more specific terms, they aim not to say what they believe to be false or for which they lack adequate evidence (maxim of quality), they aim to achieve the right level of informativeness for the purpose of the conversation (maxim of quantity), they aim to be relevant (maxim of relation) and they aim to avoid obscurity, ambiguity and wordiness of expression (maxim of manner).

Stated as such, it may at first seem that the cooperative principle and its maxims are rules of how people ought to behave in conversation. And we can immediately notice that people do not necessarily observe the maxims. They do, for instance, tell lies, give too much or too little information or produce ambiguous utterances for specific purposes. What are the maxims, then, and what is their purpose? Their purpose is to explain how contextual meaning comes about and more precisely how implicatures come about. Let us then consider how Grice views meaning and what implicatures are.

Grice's maxims and implicatures

Implicature can be defined as a meaning that cannot be worked out on the basis of the linguistic expression alone. This does not, however, mean that all such meanings are implicatures (for example, presupposition, see Grundy, 1995; explicatures, see below and Sperber and Wilson, 1995). Let us begin by outlining Grice's view of meaning and see where implicatures fit in:

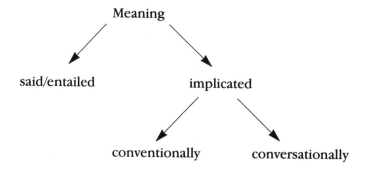

According to Grice, the *said/entailed meaning* equates to linguistic meaning and conversational maxims (or contextual information) are not needed when working out these meanings (see below, relevance theory). The *implicated meanings* are meanings beyond the words themselves, and, as can be seen from the above diagram, there are two types of implicated meanings. The *conventionally implicated meanings* do not involve the maxims but the additional meaning comes about from the meanings of the individual words. In other words, we do not need to refer to context for interpretation. In the example, 'The school won the competition', the meanings 'the school entered a competition of some sort and was better than some other schools' come from the word 'won'. In this way, these kinds of meanings can be seen as part of the meaning of the word 'won' and arise in whatever context. These types of meaning have been called *conventional implicatures*. The *conversational implicatures* are, then, the meanings that require the maxims to operate.

Maxim of quantity

The utterance 'I have two apple trees in my garden' can carry the additional meaning or implicature 'and no more'. This implicature does not arise from the words themselves, but rather from the fact that the speaker is assumed to give the right amount of information and not more or less (that is, the maxim of quantity). Note also how the speaker could be accused of purposely misleading the listener if on another occasion s/he declared that s/he had six apple trees in her/his garden. The speaker did not on the surface state that s/he had only two apple trees, but because of the maxim of quantity, the listener can rightfully assume that the implicature 'only/not more' is valid. In other words, the listener can assume that the speaker is being cooperative and in this particular example, the listener assumes that the speaker is adhering to the maxim of quantity.

Maxim of quality

The utterance 'This is really clever' can have the implicature 'this is really stupid', depending on the context. The 'implicature' comes about by the listener assuming that the speaker is upholding the cooperative principle and the maxim of quality (that is, making a truthful statement in the specific context). On the surface the utterance is violating the maxim of quality (that is, making a statement that cannot be true in the specific context) and hence the listener is alerted to the fact that s/he has to search for another meaning. One weakness of Grice's approach is that he does not specify how exactly the listener does decide on a specific implicature when he/she realizes that a maxim is violated.

Maxim of manner

The maxim of manner states that speakers try to avoid obscure expressions. In the following example (familiar to those with children) the parents are being purposely obscure (that is, are violating the maxim of manner) and because of this certain implicatures arise.

> Context: A mother and father and a 2-year-old child are hurrying out of their house to go on a car journey.
>
> Father: Did you bring any 'you know whats'? (1)
> Mother: Did I bring 'what'?
> Father: Any D-U-M-M-I-E-S (father spells out the word dummies) (2)
> Mother: I have them in my pocket.

On the surface of this conversation (that is, if we look at the words alone), it seems that the father is not cooperating in this conversation. In Grice's terms, he is violating the maxim of manner by being purposely obscure. The father is doing this in his first utterance by using 'you know whats' instead of the word 'dummies' and again in his second utterance by spelling out the word 'dummies' (spelling out is, of course, more obscure than stating something explicitly). Why would he be purposely obscure? And does this purposeful violation of the maxim of manner give rise to any meaning beyond the words themselves? Imagine what might have happened if the father had said 'dummies' in the first utterance. It is not difficult to see that the child would have most likely demanded one at that very moment and that the parents did not want her to have one. Perhaps they did not want her to have one until she became restless in the car. So, the father was being purposely obscure so that the child would not understand and that the mother would work out that she should not say the word 'dummies' either. Grice's view is that none of these additional interpretations (or implicatures) would have been possible had the maxim of manner not been violated. By maxim violation the listener is alerted to seek additional interpretation. How exactly the listener might do this, however, is not elaborated on by Grice.

Maxim of relation

This maxim simply states that speakers aim to produce relevant contributions. Let us see how this maxim can be seen operating in the following example.

> Context: A speech and language therapist (T) and a child (6;5) with communication difficulties converse.

> T: Why were you so tired this morning? You looked all sleepified.
> C: I know. I've been to Blackpool last night. (1)
> T: Oh I see.
> C: And I came back 12 o'clock. (2)
> T: Oh no wonder you're half asleep.

> (Example from Smith and Leinonen, 1992:271)

If we focus on the child's answers (1) and (2) to the adult's question 'Why were you so tired this morning?', according to Grice's theory, the two answers violate, on the surface, the maxim of relation. That is, if we interpret the two utterances linguistically (without bringing any information from our world knowledge to bear on the interpretation), then the child's utterances simply state that he had been to Blackpool the night before and he had come back at 12 o'clock. They do not state explicitly how these events connect with his being tired the next morning. But the therapist is (as are most people) clearly able to 'fill in' the gaps to arrive at some such additional meanings, as Blackpool must be a reasonable distance away from where the child lives, and needs to be travelled to, which takes time and is likely to be tiring for a small child and also he did not get back home until 12 o'clock at night, which is late for a small child. Grice's point is that these additional meanings come about first by the realization that the maxim of relation is being violated and then by the listener's need to look for another meaning so that the conversation remains cooperative and so that the maxim of relation is upheld. How precisely the listener gets from the realization of the fact that the maxim is violated to the implicatures is not, however, clear.

Exercise 7.1

Here are two small conversations. Your task is to work out what Grice's theory would have to say about how the misinterpretation in conversation A and the implicatures in conversation B arise.

Example A:

> A: I cannot get rid of this virus.
> B: Have you seen the doctor.
> A: No, it's a computer virus.

Example B:

> A: Is Mary a good cook?
> B: Do you like eating cardboard?

Comment 7.1

Example A:

B has misinterpreted A's utterance. In Grice's terms, B has assumed that A is being cooperative and hence that A is giving the right amount of information and not too much or too little given the particular context (that is, the assumption is that A is abiding by the maxim of quantity). But A's utterance was obviously not giving the right amount of information for it to be possible for B to arrive at the intended interpretation. The right amount of information would have been 'I cannot get rid of this virus in my computer'. Hence, A's first utterance can be said to violate the maxim of quality.

Example B:

B's utterance is likely to mean 'Mary is not a good cook'. How do we get to this interpretation when B's actual utterance does not say this at all? In fact, B's utterance is another question, rather than an answer, and a seemingly irrelevant one at that. According to Grice's theory, B's utterance is not a cooperative utterance as it violates the maxim of relation. On the surface, B's utterance is irrelevant, which then alerts the listener to look for a relevant interpretation in order to uphold the cooperative principle.

* * * * * *

As these examples show, according to Grice's theory, implicatures can come about by either the speaker violating or observing the maxims. What the maxims do is alert the listener to the fact that the interpretation cannot be arrived at by interpreting the linguistic expression alone. What the maxims do not, however, do is tell us what exactly happens after this realization: through what processes does the listener then work out the implicated meanings? As we will see later, relevance theory has something more workable to say about this.

Grice's theory addresses non-literal meaning too. It maintains that to arrive at an interpretation of an expression such as 'The tree is weeping', the listener realizes that this is a blatant falsehood, as we know the world, and hence the maxim of quality is violated, which in turn alerts the listener to look for interpretation somewhere else than the surface expression. How exactly this is then achieved is not addressed by Grice.

Features of implicatures

Levinson (1983) discusses five defining features of implicatures, three of which we feel are particularly important for thinking about children's pragmatic difficulties. First, implicatures can be said to be 'cancellable'. This means that the addition of some further information into the original utterance can lead to the original implicature becoming cancelled. In conversation B in Exercise 7.1, above, we said that the implicature that arises from B's utterance is that Mary is not a good cook. Imagine now that after B uttered the utterance and A worked out the implied meaning B produced a facial or some other non-verbal expression which indicated that he was only joking. This additional information would then cancel the original implicature and would produce another implicature (namely that Mary is a good/reasonable cook). Similarly, it would be possible to cancel the implicature 'I have two apple trees in my garden and not more' by simply adding 'if not more' to the original utterance. The interesting point about cancellability is that cognitive flexibility is required from the processor of language in order to be able to revise one's interpretations as new information becomes available. Those children who lack flexibility in thinking could find this aspect of pragmatic meaning difficult.

The second feature of implicatures, that of non-detachability, concerns the way in which an implicature is attached to the semantic content of an utterance rather than its linguistic form. To put this another way, the intended implicature cannot be cancelled by simply changing the linguistic form of the original utterance. Let us look at Example 7.1 again and B's utterance 'Do you like eating cardboard?' The changing of the original utterance to something like 'Cardboard sandwiches can be delicious with ketchup.' or 'She tries very hard' does not alter the implicature (that is, 'Mary is not a good cook'). This then shows how implicatures are tied to specific contexts rather than the form of words. This is not, however, true for implicatures that arise from the maxim of manner, where the form is all important. If we changed the spelled out version of 'dummies' in our example above to a non-spelled out version of the word 'dummies', the implicature would become cancelled.

The third feature that we wish to mention here is 'indeterminacy'. What this means is that we cannot be entirely sure that we have worked out the intended implicature. One utterance can potentially give rise to more than one implicature (cf. relevance theory) and hence working out implicatures is an uncertain undertaking. It involves weighing up available evidence in order to come up with the most likely interpretation (see also Chapter 6). Again, cognitive flexibility is required in order for one to be able to engage in such a weighing up process.

Relevance theory

Throughout the above discussion of Grice's theory, reference was made to certain failings of the cooperative principle: namely, that it does not tell us how one gets from the realization that a maxim has been observed or violated to the implicature. Although recognizing the importance of Grice's work, Sperber and Wilson (1995) question the need for all the maxims in order to explain how pragmatic meaning comes about. In fact they propose that the maxims could be reduced to just one: the principle of relevance. It is not within the scope of this chapter to go into the detailed arguments put forward by Sperber and Wilson, but we will simply note two of their points here (see also Wilson and Sperber, 1981).

(1) Grice's maxims are not explicit enough. They do not specify how exactly one gets from the linguistic meaning to the implicated meaning. For instance, the maxim of relation simply states 'Be relevant'. To what? How? What is it to be relevant?

(2) Contrary to Grice, Sperber and Wilson believe that pragmatic principles (and specifically the principle of relevance) have a role to play in the 'said' (=linguistic meaning). For instance, sentences that have words with multiple meanings need to be disambiguated before implicatures can be worked out. In other words, we need to work out whether 'orange' in the sentence 'Add orange to it' means 'orange juice' or 'a colour' before we can begin to work out what might be implicated by the utterance. In addition to disambiguation, a referent needs to be assigned to 'it' in the above sentence. It is believed that in both disambiguation and reference assignment the principle of relevance is involved as we need to bring the context to bear into the interpretation process. We will return to this below.

The principle of relevance states that every ostensive piece of communication carries a guarantee of optimal relevance. By ostensive communication Sperber and Wilson (1995) mean communication that makes intention to communicate manifest (or evident). In other words, every act of communication that is intended to be communicative guarantees to the listener that it is *optimally relevant* to him/her as has been *judged by the speaker*. What exactly does this mean? (see also Leinonen and Kerbel, 1999).

Sperber and Wilson believe that information is optimally relevant to the hearer if it interacts in certain ways with previous knowledge to produce an outcome with the least possible processing effort. This feels intuitively valid in that it captures and explains the situation where one does not understand another person's contribution because what is said does not connect with anything else that one knows (for example, a discussion on astrophysics would be lost on many). What is suggested, then, is that both language production and language comprehension are about making connections between what has been said and what is known. Furthermore, as any one linguistic expression can have a number of possible interpretations, how is it that we choose the intended one? According to the principle of relevance we choose the one we can arrive at with the least possible processing effort. Sperber and Wilson suggest that we go for the first possible interpretation (= least processing effort) which has adequate contextual support (in Sperber and Wilson's terms, an expression that has an adequate range of contextual or cognitive effects).

Following Wilson and Sperber (1981), we have constructed the following example to illustrate what is meant by the interaction of information when we comprehend utterances. Please note that this is not intended to be an example of real communication, but an example that illustrates a number of possibilities in one example. In this example, B1–B4 are different answers to the question posed by 'A':

A: Did your daughter get a place at the nursery school?
B1: No, she did not get a place at the nursery school.
B2: You had to put your child's name down last term to get a place at the nursery school.
    I did not put my daughter's name down last term.
B3: I did not put my daughter's name down last term.
    (shared knowledge: You had to put your child's name down last term to get a place.)
B4: I did not put my daughter's name down last term. (no shared information)

The question we need to ask here is how is it that the answers B1, B2, B3 and B4 are all taken by the listener to mean 'No, my daughter did not get a place at the nursery school.' How do we get to this interpretation?

To realize that B1 is a relevant answer to A, the linguistic meaning of B1 is important in working out its relevance (but see also explicatures, reference assignment and enrichment below). There is no need to go much beyond the linguistic meaning as there are no implicatures involved but what is actually said gives us most of the answer to the question.

To understand that B2 is a relevant answer to A, we need to deduce, by rules of logic, from what is explicitly said that B's daughter did not get a place at the nursery school. Now the answer is not simply in the linguistic expressions themselves (as in B1). The two utterances act as two premises on the basis of which the conclusion (that is, the implied meaning) is drawn.

> Premise 1: You had to put your child's name down last term to get a place at a nursery school.
> Premise 2: I didn't put my daughter's name down last term.
> Conclusion: My daughter did not get a place at a nursery school.

The point here is that to arrive at the implicature we need to engage in a deductive process (see also Chapter 6).

B3 is different from B1 and B2 in that the utterance alone is not sufficient for rendering the answer relevant to the question. The hearer needs to access the shared knowledge from his/her memory (that is, you had to put your child's name down last term) which then acts as a premise (as Premise 1 above), together with the given verbal information, in a deduction process. Here we have given verbal information interacting with previous knowledge to produce an outcome (the intended implicature) and it is this interaction which enables the relevance of the utterance to be proven (= the utterance to be understood).

Finally, to prove the relevance of B4 to A, the hearer needs to construct a premise (you had to put your child's name down last term to get a place; Premise 1, above) on the basis of his or her world knowledge and then use this and the given verbal information as the two premises in the deduction process. Again, the outcome of this process is the intended implicature.

We can make *five points* with this example:

(1) Sperber and Wilson believe that working out the relevance of an utterance involves the process of deduction (as exemplified in this chapter, but see also strengthening of assumptions and elimination of assumptions in Sperber and Wilson, 1995). But they also believe that

inferential communication is essentially an uncertain process where listeners can construct assumptions only on the basis of the evidence provided. Even in the best of conditions, communication can fail, because it is essentially guessing, but not random guessing, since we have the principle of relevance to guide us. Hence, the process of deduction does not give a guarantee that the intended meaning will be worked out. The point that Sperber and Wilson make is that although deduction plays a central role in discerning meaning, the comprehension process itself is still inductive (uncertain) in nature and the uncertainty surfaces when we have to bring information from the context (including world knowledge) into the deduction process.

(2) The process of deduction, together with the concept of processing effort, renders relevance a central aspect of human cognition. It is further believed that inferential comprehension involves central cognitive processes rather than specialized mechanisms, as would be involved in, say, perceptual or linguistic processing. Hence, comprehension (and production) of pragmatic meaning and cognition are intrinsically linked. Furthermore, cognitive factors such as speed of processing, complexity of input and accessibility of information from memory have an effect on one's ability to work out the relevance of an utterance (= one's ability to understand or produce utterances).

(3) Relevance involves interaction of what is stated with one's world (including shared) knowledge to produce pragmatic implications (implicatures). This interaction may involve accessing and/or constructing of premises. The former can be considered cognitively less taxing than the latter.

(4) Working out implicatures is a 'two-step' process: it involves working out (an) implicated premise(s) (that is, either accessing shared knowledge or constructing a premise) and then on the basis of this the intended meaning through the process of deduction.

(5) We may ask how it is that we come to access the particular information needed for working out the intended meanings and not some other information. This is where the principle of relevance guides us to the interpretation that has the greatest contextual support which can be arrived at with the least processing effort.

We hinted in the above example that before implicatures can be worked out the principle of relevance may have a role to play in working out 'the linguistic meaning' too. Let us consider this further. If someone came to a room, and simply said 'That film was excellent', and those hearing this utterance had no knowledge of any film, the hearers could not comprehend this utterance beyond the words themselves (would only comprehend it 'linguistically'). That is, they would not be able to take the conversation any further (for example, by saying 'I thought it was rubbish'). In Sperber and Wilson's terms they would not be able to comprehend it propositionally (because they cannot assign the appropriate reference for 'that film'), which we need to be able to do in communication.

A central part of relevance theory is the notion of an *explicature*. This is a meaning which is in between the linguistic meaning (or non-propositional logical form, in Sperber and Wilson's terms) and implicatures. For instance, to be able to begin to work out any implicated meanings of the expression 'It's time to put down the baby' it is first necessary to disambiguate the meaning of 'put down' as meaning either 'put to bed' or 'kill/let die(!)'. The meaning chosen on the basis of *disambiguation* (or other such process, see below) is called an explicature. But how is it that one chooses the former meaning rather than the latter? The first interpretation allowed by the principle of relevance is the 'put to bed' meaning since this is the only viable interpretation in the context of babies given the state of the world. Even in a hospital context, a doctor is highly unlikely to use such an insensitive expression if, say, a baby's life support was to be switched off. After working out the explicature, it is then possible to work out implicatures such as 'please hand the baby back to me', 'can you not see the baby is very tired, it's time you stopped bouncing him/her on your knee', 'Don't ever touch my baby again'.

Linguistic meaning is viewed by Sperber and Wilson in terms of a specialized linguistic processor which produces non-propositional logical forms. These are semantically incomplete forms that are not capable of being true or false. A sentence such as 'He stepped on her foot' cannot be true or false as it stands. It needs to undergo *reference assignment* first, to fill in the conceptually empty slots 'he' and 'her' before it becomes capable of being true or false (propositional). The outcome of this 'filling in process' is called an explicature. So, linguistic meaning can be said to be non-propositional and explicatures propositional.

In addition to disambiguation or reference assignment, an explicature can come about through *enrichment*. This is a process that enriches or expands a non-propositional form to a propositional form (that is, a semantically incomplete form to a semantically complete form). In the following example,

A: What did you get for your birthday? (1)
B: A new watch. (2)
A: Spoilt. (3)
B: Just a bit. (4)

Utterances (1), (2), (3) and (4) need to be enriched by the listeners into full propositional forms (= explicatures) corresponding to something like the following before they can be understood:

(1) 'What presents did you, B, receive for your birthday?'
(2) 'I, the speaker B, was given as a present a new watch for my birthday.'
(3) 'You, the listener B, are overindulged by receiving such a nice present.'
(4) 'I, the speaker B, agree with you, the listener A, that getting a new watch constitutes spoiling to quite a large extent.'

The enriching or expanding follows the principle of relevance so that the most contextually relevant explicatures requiring the least possible processing effort are worked out. For instance, in (2) above we would not expand the utterance to 'I want to buy a new watch' in this context.

The notion of an explicature adds an important dimension to meaning and, as Grundy (1995) points out, it can be viewed as an additional point in the comprehension (or production) process at which a person can experience difficulty. More precisely, Grundy hypothesizes that communication can break down at any of the following levels:

Linguistic meaning (non-propositional logical form)
Explicatures (propositional)
Implicated premises
Implicated conclusions (implicatures)

It is clear that being able to break down the language comprehension/production process into such components is potentially much more useful than simply stating that a child has difficulty with the comprehension and/or production of pragmatic meaning.

EXERCISE 7.2

Why is A's answer considered relevant to B's question in the following example? In other words, how do we get from the actual answer to the intended meaning 'Peter was not invited to John's birthday party'? Your task is first to work out the explicature and then the implicated premise and implicated conclusion (implicatures).

A: Was Peter invited to John's birthday party?
B: Peter is not John's good friend.

Comment 7.2

According to relevance theory, to get from the actual utterance to the intended one, the following 'steps' would need to take place:

Step 1: *Explicature*: Peter, a male person known to both A and B, is not a good friend of John, a male person known to both A and B.

Step 2: *Implicated premise*: Only John's good friends were invited to his birthday party.

Step 3: *Implicated conclusion*: Peter was (therefore) not invited to John's birthday party (= intended meaning).

EXERCISE 7.3

Here are some statements about relevance theory which explore some of the basic concepts we have introduced above. Your task is to say whether the claims made in the statements are *valid* or *invalid* and why.

(1) An utterance is optimally relevant if it produces in the listener's mind the meanings intended by the speaker with the least possible processing effort by the listener.

(2) The cognitive process of inferencing is central to relevance.

(3) Deduction plays no role in the comprehension of implicatures, since the comprehension process is essentially inductive in nature.

(4) The processes of enrichment, disambiguation and reference assignment are involved in working out implicatures.

(5) There is more than one possible explicature for the following utterance: 'I brought you up.'

(6) Comprehension difficulty can be experienced at various points in the comprehension process.

Comment 7.3

(1) This is a *valid* statement. It states the principle of relevance.

(2) This is *valid* since to work out the relevance of an utterance (that is, to understand it) the listener needs to be able to connect it with his/her previous knowledge/world knowledge. This connecting involves the interaction of given information with known information (that is, previous/world knowledge) and involves the cognitive process of inferencing (namely, deduction).

(3) This is *invalid*. While it is true that comprehension is inductive in the sense that there are many possible interpretations, Sperber and Wilson believe that when working out the relevance of an utterance

(as in 2 above) the process of deduction is used. The principle of relevance decides which interpretation is chosen in any particular context.

(4) This is *valid*. These processes are involved in arriving at explicatures, which are then used for working out implicatures.

(5) This is *valid*. The utterance needs to undergo reference assignment with regard to the words 'I' and 'you' and disambiguation for the phrase 'brought up'. Two 'levels' of disambiguation are needed here. First, through syntactic disambiguation, following the principle of relevance, we need to determine whether 'brought up' is a phrasal verb or a verb plus a preposition (for example, 'bring the parcel up'). Let us assume that the context suggests the former. Then, lexical disambiguation is called for to choose between the meanings 'to care for/rear', 'to mention' or 'to vomit'. Again, disambiguation occurs through the principle of relevance, which in the context of a father talking to his son would yield the first interpretation of the ambiguous phrase.

(6) This is *valid*. Relevance theory suggests different 'points' at which comprehension can break down and it may well be that breakdown at certain points rather than others suggests different degrees of severity of a problem.

One important point to consider in the clinical context is that optimal relevance involves the speaker making judgements about the hearer's cognitive abilities and contextual resources (including their ability to use world knowledge and other contextual information in interpretation). This, then, means that the speaker can overestimate or underestimate the hearer's resources, resulting in potential communication difficulties. Overestimation would result in a listener's inability to interpret intended implicatures, and underestimation would result in undue spelling out of information which could be assumed to be known by the listener. It is then clear that theory of mind difficulties would result in pragmatic language difficulties.

This relevance theory account of the language comprehension/ production process suggests the following about pragmatic impairment in children:

(1) Difficulties which are sometimes thought of as semantic (for example, ambiguity, ellipsis, pronouns) are now squarely placed within the domain of pragmatics, since the principle of relevance is involved in working out the propositional content of utterances. In other words, the principle of relevance has a role to play in working out the explicit meaning of utterances (that is, explicatures). Semantic deficits would

then involve difficulty with the acquisition of non-propositional meaning (linguistic meaning). Given this clearer delineation of semantics and pragmatics, it should now be easier to determine whether a particular communication breakdown occurs at the level of semantics or pragmatics.

(2) Pragmatic breakdown can occur at various (potentially testable) points in the comprehension/production process. The first possibility is that a child has difficulty explicating the linguistic meaning into a propositional meaning by enrichment, reference assignment or disambiguation. In this case, pragmatic breakdown occurs at the level of explicature, which then blocks the possibility of working out implicatures. The second possibility is that the breakdown occurs at the point of working out implicated premises. In this case, a further differentiation can be made of a breakdown in retrieving existing information as a premise or constructing new premises on the basis of existing information. The latter may be cognitively more taxing than the former. Finally, pragmatic breakdown can occur at the point of an implicated conclusion, whereby either the child is not able to use the process of deduction to arrive at the conclusion or the child is not able to weigh up the available evidence to arrive at the most relevant conclusion (the principle of relevance would not be working appropriately here).

Developmental notes

So far, relevance theory has been applied only minimally to the study of child language. We are able to comment on two studies here which have explored normal child language acquisition within this theoretical perspective. Kiss (1996) raises a number of important points in a discussion paper on theory of mind research, cognitive development and acquisition of pragmatic competence from relevance theory perspective. When and how, for instance, does intentional communication appear and what kinds of behaviours would indicate the presence of 'ostensive-inferential' communication? When and how does informative intention (to inform the listener of something) and communicative intention (to inform the listener of one's informative intention) emerge? When and how does a child acquire the principle of relevance? In asking this final question, Kiss recognizes Sperber and Wilson's (1987) view that the principle of relevance need not be learned but applies without exception. Kiss is of the view, however, that this unnecessarily avoids 'hard questions about the acquisition and learnability of this principle' (p.137).

An exploration by Foster-Cohen and Konrad (1996) showed how relevance theory was able to explain the use and structure of conditionals used by adults in interactions with children. On the basis of their data of 98 parent-to-child conditionals, they argued that even small children (4½ -year-olds) interpret irony and sarcasm expressed by conditionals, when they are assumed to be too young to be able to do so. This is because the content of the conditionals so clearly violates the children's contextual beliefs that in order to uphold the assumption of relevance, they are forced to draw an implicature. The kinds of conditionals that are referred to here are of the type 'It's really burning hot so if you would like to burn your mouth feel free'. Foster-Cohen and Konrad argue that these kinds of conditionals with outrageous consequences 'involve a clear violation of background assumptions which forces the interpretation that the parent cannot be truthful' (p.146). They further conclude that 'once children have a theory of mind (however elementary) relevance kicks in, because rationality kicks in' (p.147) and that young children's difficulties in interpreting implicatures reflect their smaller contextual resources (that is, the fact that they have less world experience) and adults' difficulties in assessing children's contextual resources (that is, adults may have difficulty knowing what the child knows and is able to bring to the interpretation process).

Some work has been done in the context of foreign language learning within the relevance theory perspective. Grundy (1995) reports on his exploration of foreign language learners' comprehension of jokes and demonstrates the usefulness of this approach in pinpointing where in the comprehension process the failure to get the joke occurs. For instance, disambiguation may be required for the joke to come off.

Clinical populations

Again, relevance theory has been applied only minimally to the exploration of communication difficulties in children. We will report on three pieces of work here: Happé's studies of comprehension of non-literal meaning by autistic children (1993, 1994, 1995) and Leinonen and Kerbel's (1999) exploration of communication difficulties of pragmatically impaired children.

Happe's (1993) starting point was that theory of mind deficits in autism reflect a relationship between a degree of deficit (failure in all theory of mind tasks, failure in first- and second-order tasks or failure in second-order tasks only) and the ability to understand language which expresses a thought either literally (that is, 'Father was very very cross, he really was angry') or metaphorically ('Father was very very cross, he really was a volcano'). Irony was deemed to require the most sophisticated theory of mind abilities, followed by metaphor. All autistic children were expected to perform equally on the literal conditions (synonym and simile conditions). The results confirmed that, indeed, the autistic individual's ability to comprehend language related to their theory of mind abilities, as predicted. Interestingly, however, the highest functioning subgroup of children (in terms of theory of mind) who performed well in all the language comprehension tasks (including irony) had difficulty in understanding language in everyday communicative situations (Happé, 1994), suggesting that the more open-ended contextual and processing demands may compound with theory of mind difficulties in communication.

According to relevance theory, all utterances, which are intended to be communicative, are interpreted as manifestations of speakers' intentions (and thoughts). Hence, one would expect autistic individuals with theory of mind deficits to have difficulty with comprehension of intentions and motivations behind all utterances (for example, joke; persuasion). Happé (1994) showed that the three groups of autistic individuals with differing theory of mind abilities (as in Happé, 1993, above) were discriminated in terms of their abilities to give adequate explanations for utterances produced by characters in stories. Instead of attributing the appropriate motivation to the character (for example, James is joking), the lower functioning autistic individuals would find a cause in the physical world as an explanation. For instance, in order to explain why a character used a figure of speech 'a frog in your throat' one person said that the story character had swallowed a frog. Happé comes to the conclusion that the ability to comprehend intentional language in these individuals relates to their theory of mind abilities. Interestingly, however, the autistic individuals used mental state words as much as control subjects (for example, think: x is joking) in their answers but these were used inappropriately in the specific story contexts. This could, then, suggest that the individuals had the ability to attribute mental states to others, but in the context of story comprehension and everyday communication where complex processing demands are placed on individuals and where the principle of relevance needs to kick in they fail to attribute appropriate mental states and intentions, not necessarily because of theory of mind difficulties, but because of other cognitive difficulties.

In their discussion paper on relevance theory and pragmatic impairment, Leinonen and Kerbel (1999) use data to show how the theory offers a way of explaining why, in a given context, a particular language expression is problematic. They show how the theory enables one to pinpoint where in the production and comprehension process breakdown occurs (for example, at the level of explicature or implicature) and why (for example, the process of enrichment is not working appropriately). The data exploration shows, for instance, that a child may have difficulty producing relevant answers to questions because s/he may have worked out an explicature which is different from the one intended. It is further shown that difficulty with the process of enrichment can account for such explicature failures. If a child fails to work out appropriate explicatures then comprehension of implicatures is blocked, since explicatures act as premises in the inference process that is needed for working out the implicatures. This in turn would suggest that the principle of relevance is not working appropriately or is only working up to a point. In this way the theory moves us away from a mere description of surface behaviours to a better understanding of how communication difficulty at a particular point in time comes about. It also enables one to explore how and why whole conversations may be failing or not moving in desired directions and how certain kinds of contributions by others may be more facilitative than others. The paper also makes a number of methodological points, advocating both qualitative and quantitative paradigms as useful when working with relevance theory. The theory also suggests a close connection between pragmatic and cognitive (dys)functioning given that relevance, and its maximization in communication, are squarely placed within human cognition. It also emphasizes the importance of world experience and experience of relationships.

Clinical data

EXERCISE 7.4

Here is a small data sample from Sarah, who is a 10-year-old child with pragmatic comprehension difficulties. Data from Sarah have also been discussed in Leinonen and Letts (1997b) and previous chapters of this book. Your task is to explore the italicized (and numbered) utterances by using the relevance theory concepts outlined in this chapter. More specifically, in relation to Sarah's utterances (1, 2, 4 and 7) please consider whether break-down occurs at the level of explicit or implicit meaning, and, if the latter, can we point to a particular process (reference assignment; disambiguation; enrichment)? Consider also whether any of this could be considered as evidence of Sarah having difficulty with the principle of relevance. In relation to the adult's utterances (3, 5 and 6), please consider what explicatures and implicatures are intended by the utterances (that is, what Sarah would need to be able to work out in order to begin to comprehend them).

S = Sarah
A = Adult (researcher; one of the authors)

The following extract is part of a longer conversation.

S: You know, after Christmas I am going on holiday.
A: Mmm

S: And I won't be at school.
A: Where are you going then?
S: I don't know. I might go to *the same holiday*. I am not going to *a different one*. (1)
A: The same as what?
S: *The same holiday.* (2) Umm we like going on the beach.
A: Umm *It'll be a bit cold in January, after Christmas, won't it?* (3)
S: Yeah. *A bit cold.* (4)
A: *Do you think that you still go on a beach holiday?* (5) Or is it – *do you have to go on an aeroplane?* (6)
S: Umm *no going on a train.* (7)
A: Going to fly? All right. So you are not coming back after Christmas to school.

This conversation is not moving in the intended direction (for A to know more about S's holiday). It is rather hard-going for both A and S. What would relevance theory say about this? Why isn't the conversation successful?

Comment 7.4

We shall comment on each numbered utterance in turn following the discussion on relevance theory presented in this chapter.

(1) When producing these two utterances, Sarah does not seem to be following the principle of relevance. She does not guarantee that the adult will be able to assign referents to the utterances 'the same holiday' and 'different one'. In other words, the adult cannot comprehend the utterances because she cannot come up with the needed 'explicature'.

(2) Sarah is not providing adequate clarification to the adult question 'The same as what?' Why might this be? We can hypothesize as follows: in order to be able to begin to provide the clarification requested by the adult, Sarah would have to enrich and disambiguate the adult's question to give the following complex explicature: 'Which holiday is the holiday you are going on identical to?' Only after being able to come up with this explicature would Sarah be able to begin to answer the question. Our hypothesis is that she may not be able to arrive at this explicature and hence she simply repeats her previous utterance in order to fulfil the obligation to take a turn. We need to look for further evidence for this hypothesis.

(3) This adult utterance carries the following intended meaning, which is not explicitly encoded in the expression: 'You cannot go on a beach holiday in January in this country.' (Note: to arrive at this intended

meaning/implicature an explicature will also have to be worked out: 'The weather will be too cold in January, after Christmas, for you to go on a beach holiday in this country'; the linguistic expression has undergone the processes of reference assignment; disambiguation; enrichment.)

(4) Sarah's answer 'yeah, a bit cold' indicates that she has not comprehended the intended meaning/implicature. It may well be that she has not worked out the explicature either, without which there is no chance of comprehending or challenging the implicature (cf. Step 3 in the comprehension process). We cannot tell from this example whether she has worked out the explicature, but from the utterance (2), above, we could hypothesize that she has not (albeit that working out the explicature is likely to be more complicated in 2 than in this utterance). What Sarah's answer suggests here more strongly, we could argue, is that she may be comprehending at the level of linguistic meaning by simply reacting to the words, and hence echoing the words 'bit cold' from the adult utterance.

(5) This adult utterance is intended to be interpreted as follows (carries the following implicature): 'You cannot go on a beach holiday in this country in January', for which the explicature 'Do you, Sarah, believe that you, Sarah and family, will go on a beach holiday despite the cold?' will first have to be worked out.

(6) This adult utterance has the intended meaning (implicature): 'You can of course go on a beach holiday outside this country in January', for which the following explicature would have to be worked out '"Do you, Sarah and family, go on an aeroplane to your beach holiday?'

(7) Sarah's answer here indicates that she has not comprehended at the level of the intended meaning (implicature). This is further supported by the fact that her answer 'going on a train' confirms the adult's initial assumption that Sarah was going on a beach holiday in the UK. The answer would indicate that Sarah has comprehended at the level of explicature (note how this answer is not an echo as could be suggested in case of utterance 4, 'a bit cold').

Linguistic interpretation

In Chapter 6 we noted that Sarah may have difficulty with comprehension of inferential meaning. Having now looked at Sarah's pragmatic skills from a relevance theory perspective, albeit using a very small data sample, we are in a position to make more specific hypotheses about Sarah's communication difficulties.

The data exploration would suggest the following. Sarah has difficulty with comprehension of implicatures. She does not show in her answers that she has grasped that the adult is trying to say, in many different ways, that it is not very likely for Sarah to go on a beach holiday in January in the UK. It is not possible to tell from these data whether Sarah has problems with the construction of implicated premises and/or with the working out of implicated conclusions. As we will explore below, Sarah may not get as far as implicatures, since the process may be blocked at the point of working out the intended explicatures.

The data suggest that Sarah is able to work out explicatures, but may not work out the ones intended by the adults. Leinonen and Kerbel (1999) give another example of how this happens in conversations with Sarah. In this example the adult is asking Sarah a question while they are looking at a picture of a flood scene. In this picture people have been caught unawares by a severe flood. There are various household items, cows and people clinging to bits of wood floating in the water. There are also people on the roofs of their cars.

> A: Why are people sitting on the roofs of their cars?
> S: Umm – er (laughs) – er – because because they might slip down because they might slip into the water they might slip

The adult question asks for the following explicature to be worked out: 'Why are the people in the picture sitting on the roofs of their cars rather than sitting in their cars or walking on the street?' To this question the expected answer is something like: 'because otherwise they would drown or get wet or because they are frightened'. Indeed, normally functioning 6- and 8-year-old children gave these kinds of answers in the study of Leinonen and Letts (1997b). Sarah's answer seems to be an answer to a different explicature: 'Why are the people in the picture sitting on the roofs of their cars rather than standing on the roofs of their cars?'. In this context, Sarah's answer would be sensible and appropriate (that is, 'They are sitting on the roofs of their cars rather than standing, because if they were standing they would slip into the water but because they are sitting they won't'). This example would also suggest that Sarah is capable of working out explicatures but may work out ones that are not appropriate in the particular context. Similar interpretations are possible of data presented elsewhere on pragmatically impaired children (Bishop and Adams, 1992; Mills, Pulles and Witten, 1992; Smith and Leinonen, 1992; Leinonen, 1995).

The question is, then, what is it that directs one to work out the intended explicatures? According to the theory of relevance, the principle of relevance would have this role in communication. It would direct one to work out the most contextually relevant explicature which would require the least processing effort. We would then suggest that, for some reason, the principle of relevance would not be working appropriately in these examples. This may be linked to lack of, or difficulty in accessing and/or operating with, world knowledge. Lack of linguistic knowledge (for example, lack of knowledge of multiple meanings) and theory of mind difficulties could also contribute towards an inappropriately functioning principle of relevance. In Exercise 7.4 Sarah has difficulty providing adequate information for the adult to assign referents in the utterances 'the same holiday' and 'a different one', which could be interpreted in relation to theory of mind difficulties. Interestingly, Sarah does not show difficulty with the comprehension of pronouns, but has shown problems with time deixis (Leinonen and Kerbel, 1999).

Exploration of this small data sample from Sarah shows that working within a theoretical model, such as relevance theory, is potentially more useful than simply saying that Sarah has problems with pragmatic meaning. We are able to generate hypotheses that can be examined further by both qualitative and empirical methods.

As Leinonen and Kerbel (1999) further point out, working within a theoretical framework renders appropriacy judgements more reliable because we are guided by the theory rather than by our 'intuitions' and sociocultural norms.

Finally, it is worth noting that in the comments to the data in Exercise 7.4, we suggested that some explicatures may be easier (or more difficult) to work out than others. This would presumably be true of implicatures too. There may be many possible reasons for this, which we will not elaborate on here, but we would simply like to note that Sperber and Wilson's (1995) notion of 'weak and strong communications' would be relevant here. Weak communications are utterances in contexts which suggest more than one possible interpretation (that is, the intended interpretation is more difficult to work out) whereas strong communications are utterances where the context strongly suggests one interpretation above others (that is, the intended meaning is easier to work out). This would provide one way forward for exploring pragmatic communication difficulties and, particularly, for explaining intermittency in pragmatic performance. Leinonen and Kerbel (1999) note that the children they studied did not always fail in their communications that involved pragmatic meaning. Explaining such intermittency in performance would be a big step forward in our understanding of pragmatic impairments in children.

Clinical interpretation

As has already been made clear, the application of relevance theory to clinical contexts has so far been extremely limited. This means that a certain amount of caution is necessary in interpreting clinical data, and especially in planning intervention, on the basis of relevance theory principles. It is possible, however, to make some observations.

It has already been shown how Sarah was unable to respond appropriately to some of the adult's questions in the data sample, either because she could not arrive at the correct explicature, or because she could not go from explicatures to the relevant implicature. A look at some of the adult's contributions reveals a degree of complexity, not in terms of linguistic form particularly, but in terms of cognitive demands. The suggestion of a beach holiday is followed up by a comment (plus a tag-question) about the temperature in January (3). The adult is obviously thinking about the viability of a beach holiday in cold weather, based perhaps on past experiences of cold seaside holidays or of her own requirement that a beach is only acceptable in warm weather. A child will not necessarily have the same concerns. Similarly, the adult continues to think along these lines in utterance (6), when she asks about the mode of transport, assuming that a beach holiday would be appropriate in a warmer location, but the only way to reach such a location quickly when travelling from Britain in January is by plane. Again the child is less likely to have the required experience or concerns to arrive at the correct premises here (that is, that the adult thinks there are places where a beach holiday is feasible in January, that these places are a long way away, that travel-time for a holiday may be limited so air is the best mode of transport). If these premises were not available for Sarah (and, to be sure, we would need to investigate this further), then she can be seen to be responding with sensible strategies to both the suggestion that it will be cold in January (Sarah agrees), and the query about mode of transport (by train).

In the absence of relevance theory terminology, an experienced clinician might well suggest that the adult's input is too 'high level' here. Many adults, if anxious to retrieve the situation, would try to simplify the cognitive demands of their stimuli, by breaking down the processing load. This may not necessarily be the case in the school context where the expectations of a 10-year-old, such as Sarah, are likely to motivate the kinds of questions asked of children. The issue of cold weather might be tackled by pursuing a series of questions something like the following:

What sort of thing do you do on a beach holiday?
Will you enjoy doing this if the weather is cold?

Won't the weather be cold in January?
Are you going somewhere warm to avoid the cold?

How does this fit in with the notion that listeners arrive at their interpretations of what is said according to minimal processing effort, since the processing here is evidently high? The adult has misjudged Sarah's ability to process the input, and consequently produces the complex implicatures. In other words, the listener can only arrive at the intended meaning with minimal processing effort when the one producing the language has judged correctly that the contexts (for example, knowledge and experiences) that are needed for the interpretation are indeed readily available for the listener. The listener will also need to be able to use the relevant contexts in order to arrive at the intended interpretations. The adult had not fully considered that the links between holidays, beaches, warm weather, going abroad and air travel, which are well rehearsed and obvious for an adult, may not be so for Sarah. It could, of course, be that these links are available for Sarah, but that she is not able to bring them to the interpretative context when needed. It may also be that she has difficulty taking the preceding conversation into account when processing for meaning. There are a number of possibilities why Sarah has difficulty with contextual meaning, all of which need careful further investigation.

One way in which Sarah can be helped here is to make the stimuli less demanding in terms of arriving at the correct implicatures, by making premises explicit and by working carefully through a logical sequence. In a similar way, the need to work hard at enrichment can also be diminished. It has been pointed out that the adult question 'the same as what?' in response to Sarah's suggestion that she might go to 'the same holiday', needs to be enriched to something like: 'which holiday is the holiday you are going to identical to?' This enrichment as it stands is impossibly complex grammatically and conceptually for the clinical context, as well as sounding bizarrely stilted (and not therefore a good model). It is possible, however, to enrich somewhat differently by breaking the concepts into a series of queries, along the lines of:

Have you had a holiday like this before?
Where was this holiday?
Are you planning to go to the same place this time?

The challenges for the adult in simplifying both the enrichment and the implicature processes is to keep the stimuli both cognitively and linguistically simple enough for the child to be able to cope and to try to remain alert to what the child is trying to say. The resultant interactions are likely to become somewhat long-winded, providing a further challenge of keeping the child interested. A more extreme example of the type of situation where this is very difficult is that of interacting with an adult who had an acquired dysphasia of the Wernicke's type. Here comprehension of language may be severely impaired, but expression remains fluent. As a result of poor self-monitoring and paraphrasic errors, however, the dysphasic adult's output is difficult to follow. Requests for clarification (comparable to those suggested to enrich the 'same holiday' example above) tend to be poorly understood by the dysphasic adult who then answers with a similarly confusing response which then itself requires enrichment and clarification. Somewhat counterintuitively, therapists working with such cases need to keep all input simple and to the point and to avoid getting distracted by doomed attempts at clarification. This is plainly not the case with children like Sarah, although such problems may arise if the child has a severe comprehension problem. Except in such cases, the adult interactant here is working with comparatively better linguistic ability than the child, but must be aware of the cognitive loads and the interpretative contexts being imposed.

In addition to modifying input in the ways suggested above, there might be specific activities that can be carried out with the child to help him/her to maximize abilities in various subcomponents of 'relevance'. Work on referring expressions, as discussed in Chapters 4 and 6, should help the child both to assign reference accurately and to make reference assignment maximally possible for the listener. To aid disambiguation, it may be useful to encourage the child to become more aware of the possibilities of lexical items having multiple meanings. An assessment procedure sometimes used with school-age language impaired children is to ask them to think of as many meanings as they can for a word. A frequent pattern is that having accessed one meaning, the child finds it difficult to shift to a completely different one. However, after a few attempts and examples from the therapist, they may realize that this is possible and go on to do further items successfully. In these cases it may be less the case that the child does not initially understand the task, but that s/he has never considered words in this way. Of course, in this task words are presented out of context, and in real-life situations the choice of meaning is heavily contextually determined in on-line processing conditions. It has been suggested that children with pragmatic deficits find processing in open-ended conversational contexts more taxing than in more well-defined conditions (for example, Bishop and Adams, 1991).

Summary

In this chapter we have looked at two theories that aim to explore how it is that utterances can mean more than is suggested by the linguistic expression itself, and how it is that we choose a particular interpretation for an utterance rather than another. Grice's cooperative principle and its four maxims provide some valuable insight into pragmatic meaning, but the problem with this approach is that it is not explicit enough in telling us how it is that we get from what is said to what is intended. The relevance theory of Sperber and Wilson (1995), on the other hand, provides a more explicit account of how pragmatic meaning comes about. It enables one to explore comprehension and production in clinically useful terms, given particularly that difficulty can be seen to occur at various points in the comprehension and production processes. Research using this theory in the study of language and pragmatically impaired children remains to be carried out, but the clinical promise carried by this approach is enormous. If, for instance, we were to devise comprehension tests on the basis of relevance theory, we would progress in our ability to discriminate between semantic and pragmatic difficulties and we would be in a position to describe the nature of the difficulty in more precise terms. We could also target intervention more specifically given the different 'steps' involved in the comprehension and production processes.

Chapter 8: What is pragmatic impairment?

Key words: autistic syndrome/spectrum/continuum disorders, pragmatic impairment and specific language impairment, specific pragmatic impairment, cognition, research questions.

Aims

Let us start with a relatively non-controversial statement. Children exist whose communication difficulties are best *described* in pragmatic terms. We have argued that a clinically most useful description of children's pragmatic impairments would be one which has *explanatory power* (which has psycholinguistic reality). Although we are still a long way from explaining children's pragmatic difficulties, we have, however, moved forward in a number of directions. It is worth casting an eye back to the research questions put forward by McTear in 1985(c). We stated in Chapter 1 that one of our aims was to clarify our thinking with regard to McTear's points. Do we now know more about how, or indeed whether, pragmatic impairments relate to impairments at other levels of language? Are we able to say whether pragmatic impairments have socio-interactional or cognitive bases and whether they are closely related to other developmental disorders? What exactly is pragmatic impairment? Is it a unitary phenomenon or are there different subtypes? Or, indeed, does it exist at all? We also set out to explore in this book what could be rightfully called pragmatic impairment from the point of view of the field of pragmatics. How far have we progressed with these aims and have we raised any further issues?

It is not surprising that controversy surrounds pragmatic impairment. In fact, this has been inevitable for a number of reasons.

(1) Because clinicians and researchers have adopted a very wide-ranging

definition of pragmatics, pragmatic impairment has become an all-encompassing category, without clear defining features and sufficiently constrained inclusion criteria.

(2) Despite early efforts by researchers to signal to clinicians that we are not in a position to diagnose children with pragmatic impairments, clinicians have felt the real need to use pragmatic impairment (and related terms) to refer to children with certain kinds of communication difficulties (for purely practical purposes).

(3) Because of the above two points, research into children's pragmatic impairments has been at times circular and confused.

(4) Because of the need for clinicians to help children with pragmatic-type communication difficulties, the amount of knowledge that exists about such children has become exaggerated and applied in a manner which has not always been fully justified.

(5) Medical, psychological and linguistic views have become interwoven in the debate concerning the status of pragmatic impairment, and the validity of the concept has been called into question.

(6) Not enough attention seems to have been paid to the early calls for the need to differentiate between surface manifestations of pragmatic difficulty and their underlying causes. In scientific terms, a clearer line needs to be drawn between description and explanation.

Most of these reasons have been explored throughout the book, but let us now draw together some of the issues here and see what kind of a picture of pragmatic impairment emerges. With this overarching aim in mind, this chapter will discuss the following:

Key questions:
Is pragmatic impairment an autistic spectrum disorder?
Can environmental influences impair pragmatic performance?
Is pragmatic impairment related to specific language impairment?
Does pragmatic impairment exist?
Where does this leave the clinician?

Is pragmatic impairment an autistic spectrum disorder?

In an important paper which explores how pragmatic impairment could be related to autism and specific language impairment (SLI), Boucher (1998a) arrives at three possibilities: that pragmatic impairment is a subtype of autism, a subtype of SLI or a subtype of both, forming an intermediate disorder. We shall concentrate on autism here and discuss the other two options later. Boucher comes to the conclusion that 'the spectrum of subtypes' view of autism would be able to accommodate pragmatic impairment as a subtype of autism. She argues that if autism were viewed as a syndrome or a disorder of the autistic continuum (Wing, 1988) pragmatic impairment as a possible subtype could not be accommodated (see Boucher for a full discussion). The notion of a continuum supposes different profiles for individual children which reflect different affected behaviours and different degrees of difficulty with these behaviours. As such, the concept captures the heterogeneity which is found among people with autism and does not accommodate discrete diagnostic entities within the continuum.

Autism is currently considered to be a constellation of different subtypes which share a set of defining features but which differ from one another in at least one feature. In DSM-IV (American Psychiatric Association, 1994) autism is characterized as one of five subcategories of 'pervasive developmental disorder', the others including Asperger's syndrome and 'pervasive developmental disorder not otherwise specified' (PDD-NOS). It is this last category which offers a potential, temporary, home for pragmatic impairment. The important point here is that to qualify for this diagnosis, pragmatic impairment would have to have the defining features of pervasive developmental disorder and would also have to differ from the others in at least one respect. We are not in a position to say whether pragmatic impairment satisfies this criterion, because we do not yet have a reasonable understanding of what characterizes pragmatic impairment itself and because there have not yet been adequate studies which compare autism and pragmatic impairment. Nor is autism itself well defined, given particularly the idea of different degrees of severity of autistic difficulty (Wing, 1988). The use of terms such as 'high-level autism' and 'mild autism' confuse the issue of where the boundaries of the different subtypes of autism are and how pragmatic impairment, and even Asperger's syndrome, relate to these milder forms of autism.

Aarons and Gittens (1987) and Wing (1988) were the first to suggest that pragmatic impairment is just another term for autism. The arguments put forward rested heavily on the notion of an autistic continuum, which was considered able to accommodate less severe forms of autism, such as pragmatic impairment. Since then Boucher (1998a) has convincingly argued that the notion of an autistic continuum cannot accommodate pragmatic impairment since the idea of multidimensional profiling suggested by the notion of a continuum does not allow for diagnostic categories (which in turn would make categorization of developmental disorders impossible). Brook and Bowler (1992) reviewed relevant research on both pragmatic impairment and autism and came up with the suggestion that the two could stem from the same fundamental cognitive and interpersonal difficulties. It is important to emphasize, however, that the review of literature carried out in Brook and Bowler's paper does not enable one to conclude that pragmatic impairment is simply autism by another name and that their hypothesis remains to be investigated (but see Shields et al., 1996a and b).

Shields and colleagues (1996a and b) suggest that their two studies provide evidence for pragmatic impairment being an autistic spectrum disorder. In one of these studies a group of pragmatically impaired children were found to perform similarly to a high-functioning autistic group on theory of mind tasks and dissimilarly to a group of children with SLI. The same pattern was found in the performance of the children on right hemisphere batteries so that the pragmatic impairment group and the autism group performed similarly on the right-hemisphere tasks in contrast with the SLI group's poor performance on left-hemisphere tasks. Do these studies provide evidence for pragmatic impairment being an autistic spectrum disorder? The theory of mind tasks require the children to think what other people think, know or intend. As the key to both comprehension and production of language is the ability to attribute intentions and knowledge to others, the link between some kind of a theory of mind ability and pragmatic performance is indisputable. From this fact, the findings of this study become inevitable, as both the autistic and the pragmatically impaired children had by definition pragmatic diffi- culties, and as theory of mind abilities by definition underpin pragmatic performance. In some ways the result is predetermined by the choice of the autistic group too. The status of high-level autistic children in the autism field itself is debatable, given that they may not share all the defin- ing features of autism (that is, the Kanner-type autism) but are more like pragmatically impaired children. An interesting finding of this study is, however, that the impairment on the tasks was milder for the pragmatic impairment group than the autistic group, which may suggest a milder form of communication deficit in the former group as compared with the latter. At least clinical opinion would support this hypothesis. A similar circularity to the theory of mind study is found in the hemispheric function study. The problem here comes from the fact that the right hemisphere is known to be associated with pragmatic functioning and, as pragmatically impaired children and autistic children both have pragmatic difficulties, they by definition have difficulty with right-hemisphere tasks. A valuable finding of these studies is that the pragmatically impaired children and the SLI children were appropriately placed in the different groups in the first instance and hence the clinical view of the children was supported by the research findings.

The problems associated with the arguments put forward by researchers in autism, including the two studies of Shields and colleagues, can be characterized by the following metaphor. Say that we were to determine whether plums and peaches were the same fruit. We could choose to focus on features that we know that they share. We could set up a study to find out whether they were round, had a skin and a stone in the middle. We would find that indeed they share these features. We could similarly choose to study whether they have the defining features of fruit and again we would find that the two types of fruit share these features. It is clear that by choosing to focus on known similarities and defining features we have already determined the outcome of our study and it is clear that this would not enable us to find an answer to the question whether the two are the same or different fruit. To investigate this question we would have to look systematically for differences between the fruit and, if it turns out that these cannot be found, then we could conclude that they are the same fruit (for the time being, given that a more refined investigative tool may emerge, which may give us a different result!). Imagine also that there was a new, unique, plum which was developed to have many of the features of peaches and imagine that we decided to have this new type of plum in the study instead of traditional plums. We would then most likely find that they shared many features with peaches, and we might come to the conclusion that the differences are so negligible that the two fruit are indeed identical. But on the basis of this study we would not be able to come to the conclusion that all plums are identical to peaches, only this one specially cultured variety.

Leaving plums and peaches aside and returning to autism and pragmatic impairment, the way forward in the autistic spectrum debate would be to look for differences and this is indeed what Boucher (1998a) urges researchers to do in her paper. To make the case that pragmatic impairment is separate from autism, we don't need to show that pragmatically impaired children are impaired in pragmatic communication (because by definition they are) and that they share this difficulty with autistic children (since by definition they do), but rather we need to investigate whether they share the other defining features of autism (namely, difficulty with social relationships as a function of impairment and rigidity of thought/obsessiveness) which from current research we cannot say whether they share or not. Boucher states that we need to show reliable similarities and differences in both symptoms and underlying causes of the two in order to establish pragmatic impairment as a subtype of autism. In order to establish pragmatic impairment as a separate entity from autism we need to show more differences than similarities between the two groups of children. The question is, however, what counts as a valid number of differences and how different do the differences need to be? It is also worth noting something that Prior and colleagues (1998) have pointed out, that there is a danger that failure at certain measures (like theory of mind tasks) has become synonymous with autistic behaviour, whereas such failure can simply reflect developmental and cognitive delay rather than the autistic disorder. As with all developmental disorders, the issue of diagnosis is further obscured by the fact that the characteristics of disorders change over time (see also Botting and Conti-Ramsden, in press).

Boucher (1998a) adds to the hypotheses concerning the relationship between autism and pragmatic impairment by predicting that pragmatic impairment will prove to be a subtype of autism. The shared features will be, she predicts, a deficit in information processing of complex experience and the ability to generate behaviour and to plan. The differentiating feature will be pragmatically impaired children's lack of a fundamental problem with intersubjectivity (socio-emotional relatedness). Unfortunately, this prediction is stated in such general terms that it is difficult to see how viable it would be as a hypothesis. Will the children have difficulty with all complex experience or only that mediated by language? The ability to generate and plan all behaviour could not be impaired in these children, so which aspects of generative ability are the likely candidates for being impaired? How would children with such impairments be differentiated from those suffering from other childhood disorders such as aphasia and schizophrenia? Would it not be a possibility that pragmatically impaired children could be more specifically impaired in the processing of information which is communicated by language? As is clear from just these few questions which Boucher's prediction brings to mind, more well-defined hypotheses are needed given the already confused state of the debate.

Bishop (1989) wrote a discussion paper asking where are the boundaries of autism, Asperger's syndrome and pragmatic impairment. The suggestion is that children can have pragmatic impairment without autistic features, but there are also points at which there is overlap. Bishop placed autism as the most 'abnormal' on the dimensions of social relationships/interests and verbal communication, whereas children with Asperger's syndrome were considered more normal on these dimensions than autistic children. Pragmatically impaired children were considered more normal on the social relationships/interests dimension than the other two groups and more able on verbal communication than autistic children but less able than Asperger's children. This conceptualization constitutes a hypothesis that remains to be tested. There are others, too, who maintain that pragmatically impaired children are qualitatively different from autistic spectrum children. Botting (1998) points out that many speech and language therapists believe that pragmatically impaired children show a different pattern of development, need different intervention and have a different prognosis from children with SLI and autistic children. This clinical finding is borne out by Bishop's recent study evaluating the Children's Communication Checklist (CCC, Bishop, 1998). Although no children with a diagnosis of autism were included in the study, two groups of children with pragmatic language impairment were identified on the basis of school information. A 'semantic-pragmatic pure' group (SP pure) displayed pragmatic communication difficulties with no autistic features, whereas an 'SP plus' group did have some possible autistic features. The 'SP pure' group were found not to 'differ from other children with SLI in terms of ratings of social relationships or unusual interests, although they were clearly differentiated in terms of their communicative behaviour' (p.886). It was also the case that the scores of the 'SP pure' and the 'SP plus' groups differed significantly on the subscale of the CCC concerned with rapport.

As has become apparent in this discussion, we are not in a position to place pragmatic impairment within the autistic spectrum or to claim it as a separate diagnostic entity. To put this in Boucher's (1998b) terms we have moved some way towards providing reliable clinical and research-based descriptions of pragmatic impairment in children and thus have identified pragmatic impairment as a candidate, albeit still rather a tentative candidate, for a diagnostic entity. To gain this status in an authoritative manual (for example, DSM-IV), what needs to be provided in addition to a reliable symptom cluster is documentation of the course (developmental progression) of the disorder together with a statement on causal mechanisms and the disorder's likely response to treatment. Needless to say, pragmatic impairment is a long way from satisfying all four criteria, if indeed it ever will. It is worth noting that most recognized developmental disorders entered into the DSM-IV manual do not in fact satisfy all of these criteria.

We may then ask why do some people seem so confident in claiming pragmatic impairment as a subtype of autism, when there is not clear evidence for this. Some of this may stem from a lack of appreciation that pragmatic impairment has been largely defined in linguistic terms and autism in medical/psychological terms (Adams, 1991) and that perhaps the two need to converge for a more informative discussion. As a concession, one sometimes hears from people working primarily with autism that there may be children who are pragmatically impaired and not autistic, but that they are rare. What may be taking place is that those professionals who are highly experienced with autism come into contact with relatively few, if any, children whose complex pragmatic difficulties do not resemble autism. There is no reason why such children would be referred to them. The incidence of this type of problem may therefore become underestimated. However, we would certainly not wish to deny the possibility that professionals working primarily with people who are language impaired might also be slow to recognize subtle similarities with autism, or that failing to do so would be unhelpful.

Can environmental influences impair pragmatic performance? This is a question to which the answer is not yet known. However, it is one that requires investigation in the context of children's pragmatic impairments and autism. Without an answer, therapists, psychologists and psychiatrists could be in danger of attributing bizarre, inappropriate or disturbed communicative behaviour in children to 'autistic spectrum disorders'. The work of Rutter and colleagues (1999) on the subject of 'quasi-autistic' behaviour in children adopted from Romanian orphanages adds urgency to this question.

Is pragmatic impairment related to specific language impairment?

As we have already mentioned above, one of Boucher's possibilities, which, however, she rejects in her prediction in the end, is that pragmatic impairment is a subtype of specific language impairment. To find evidence for such a relationship, Boucher maintains that we need to show that pragmatic impairment resembles other subtypes of SLI (that is, phonological, grammatical and semantic impairments) by involving difficulties in the acquisition of language systems while also differing from the other subtypes in reliable ways. Furthermore, the communication difficulties, social cognition impairments and other manifestations of difficulty which pragmatically impaired children may experience would need to be shown to differ from difficulties experienced by autistic children. The view that pragmatic impairment is a subtype of SLI is difficult to support on theoretical grounds. The very concept of an SLI is incompatible with the possibility of including pragmatic impairment as a sub-type. The word 'specific' implies that the impairment is specific to language functioning and indeed it subscribes to the view that language processing is largely confined to separate language module(s). Pragmatic functioning, on the other hand, is not 'specific' in this sense, and as we have discussed throughout this book, it is intrinsically linked to cognitive functioning. As such, pragmatic impairment does not, by definition, involve impairment in the language acquisition mechanism, even though such difficulty may accompany pragmatic difficulty, particularly given that language develops in a communicative context. If this context is not readily available to a child as a consequence of pragmatic difficulties then language acquisition difficulties can ensue. The point is, however, that such difficulties would be secondary to the pragmatic difficulties. It is possible that SLI and pragmatic impairment coexist as a multiple language handicap (both structure- and use-impaired), but it is not theoretically possible that pragmatic impairment would be a subtype of SLI. What is, however, possible is that pragmatic problems ensue from language acquisition problems (at all linguistic levels). That is, that pragmatic performance is affected by both receptive and expressive linguistic problems.

The above view subscribes to a strict definition of SLI. In reality, both clinically and in the literature, the term is used much more loosely to cover a range of language impairments. It has been shown that SLI may not be that 'specific' after all, but that cognitive impairments may accompany SLI (for example, Johnston and Smith, 1989; Johnston, Smith and Box, 1997). Conti-Ramsden, Crutchley and Botting (1997) point out that, as children with SLI grow older, a proportion of these children exhibit significant learning problems and that more fine-tuned testing of the children's abilities early in development may enable the detection of cognitive deficits (see also Botting and Conti-Ramsden, in press).

Research has split SLI children into subgroups on a number of grounds and, as a consequence, a wide variety of subgroups have emerged. As Conti-Ramsden, Crutchley and Botting (1997) observe, ideally the subgroups should be clinically and psychometrically valid as well as adequately characterized in terms of their linguistic behaviour. By using a battery of psychometric tests and clinical interviews (with teachers and speech and language therapists) Conti-Ramsden and colleagues categorized a group of 242 7-year-old children with SLI into six subgroups. The children were deemed to have SLI as a function of attending language units in mainstream schools. One of these subgroups included children who had semantic and/or pragmatic problems which were receptive in nature. Fifty-five of the 242 children fell into this semantic/pragmatic cluster. These children did reasonably well on all the psychometric tests except number skills. The administered tests targeted grammatical comprehension (TROG); number skills, naming/vocabulary and word reading (British Ability Scales); articulation (Goldman-Fristoe Test); information processing in a narrative (the Bus Story); and non-verbal cognition (Ravens Matrices). As there are no adequate formal tests for pragmatic functioning, it was the judgements of the clinicians which placed the children into the semantic/pragmatic group. The important point of this study is that there were children whose profiles were sufficiently different from the other SLI children on the psychometric measures which were used to place them into the cluster and that this cluster was deemed by the clinicians to be characterised by semantic/pragmatic difficulties. Pragmatic impairment can be seen to have different characteristic features from other language impairments and the clinical view of these children is a reliable indicator of their differential status. These findings do not tell us about the exact nature of the relationship between pragmatic impairment and SLI, but they nevertheless provide the first large-scale support for the existence of such children as a clinically identifiable group (see also Botting and Conti-Ramsden, in press).

Does pragmatic impairment exist?

As we said at the outset of this chapter it is generally agreed that communication difficulties of children (and adults), of various diagnostic backgrounds, can be described in pragmatic terms (for example, Rapin and Allen, 1987; 1998). The controversy begins with the suggestion that pragmatic impairment may be a bona fide diagnostic category. In other words, that it can exist as a primary deficit without the existence of other developmental disorders. As we have discussed in this chapter, there are arguments put forward to support the view that pragmatic impairment is a subgroup of autism and there are others who would argue for pragmatic impairment as a separate diagnostic group (namely Bishop and Conti-Ramsden and colleagues). There are also others who sit on the fence by trying to focus on the defining characteristics of pragmatic impairment, and methods of investigating impaired pragmatic functioning, without entering the discussion of diagnosis (for example, Vance and Wells, 1994; Leinonen and Letts, 1997b; Kerbel and Grunwell, 1998b).

Although we cannot say anything definite about the status of pragmatic impairment as a diagnostic category from the research perspective, clinical opinion supports the notion that children exist whose primary deficits are pragmatic in nature. It is our view that this opinion is relatively widespread. Such children have been rejected for the diagnosis of autism, albeit that the diagnosis of autism seems to be shifting, given labels such as 'high-level autism', 'mild autism' and 'autistic spectrum children'. There is a need to identify and classify the problems of pragmatically impaired children, whether they are a justifiable diagnostic group or not, in order for clinicians to be able to provide appropriate intervention for them. The work of Conti-Ramsden, Crutchley and Botting (1997) points a way forward for future research by highlighting the importance of using clinical, linguistic and psychometric information in the classification of language impairments, including pragmatic impairments, in children.

Finally, there is also the possibility that the key features of pragmatic impairment, yet to be identified, cover those children conventionally viewed as pragmatically impaired but in addition subsume some children felt to be more centrally SLI. Bishop et al. (in press), using micro-analysis of conversation, were able to identify a subgroup of SLI children who displayed pragmatically inappropriate responses along with a low frequency of non-verbal responses. Although this group contained the majority of children from a group previously diagnosed as pragmatically impaired (by means of teacher/therapist identification plus checklist), it also contained a similar number of children previously diagnosed as typical SLI.

Where does this leave the clinician?

Depending on how experienced clinicians are or what kind of experience they have been exposed to, the present state of knowledge about children's pragmatic impairments can leave them in a difficult position. Those who have thought through the arguments with care and have encompassed the many problem areas which remain to be clarified, can find themselves dealing, in a practical sense, with fellow professionals who, although less familiar with the arguments, feel confident as to how children's problems ought to be labelled. This can be difficult for clinicians and at times disastrous for children since unsuitable educational placement and intervention regimes can result. On the whole, however, clinicians are able to deal with both semantic and pragmatic difficulties in their clients by carefully observing and recording the behaviour of each individual and then tailoring intervention to their apparent needs. The general uncertainty as to underlying causes and mechanisms is acknowledged and it is hoped that future research will enable clinicians to improve their approach. But, in the meantime, professionals offer the best help and advice that they are able.

There is relative clarity about the fact that the communicative performance of some clients is weakest in the area of linguistic functioning. Clinicians also tend to be clear that linguistic difficulties are likely to lead to some peculiarities in an individual's pragmatic performance. It is also known that environmental factors and matters such as personal confidence can play a part in the production and resolution of pragmatic difficulties. What is at present much less clear, however, is the source of the many possible forms of pragmatic difficulty and how the difficulties relate to other developmental disorders. Yet, clinicians are not in a position to defer intervention and refuse advice and are therefore searching for reasonable assumptions on which to proceed.

In many of the clinical examples we have given in this book, it has been apparent that some of the input from the adult interlocutor has been less than helpful to the child. The adult may have failed to recognize or encourage the child's communicative intentions, perhaps because they were following their own agenda. Even where the approach is maximally facilitative, the adult may confuse the child by using pronouns and other deictic terms where the child finds it difficult to identify the referent, or the adult may use utterances that require complex enrichment or inferencing skills of the child. These characteristics of the adult input have allowed us to illustrate the sorts of problems the child is likely to encounter every day, and which therefore have an assessment value. Clinicians need, however, to be aware of how they can modify their interaction and input to aid both assessment and remediation. As regards assessment, seeing how the child responds under optimal conditions will give insight as to whether there is a true pragmatic disorder present or not. For remediation, a carefully planned programme can be developed to help the child first of all gain confidence and feel comfortable with his/her therapy interlocutor, and then to be able to cope with progressively more demanding input.

Where next?

It will not be in the immediate future that we will know what status pragmatic impairment will have among developmental disorders. Much research remains to be carried out to determine which features best identify such children and how they relate to other developmental disorders. There is a need to investigate a variety of factors, including cognitive skills, the children's understanding of cause and effect, their ability to plan and execute plans and their ability to work within the temporal confines of a conversation. How we go about doing some of this depends on the availability of methods and investigative tools. There is currently no way of testing reliably someone's conversational functioning or other pragmatic skills, but as we have hopefully demonstrated in this book, there are some useful linguistic methods available for one to gain a better understanding of children's pragmatic functioning, whether the children are specifically pragmatically impaired or not. Some of these methods would lend themselves to more targeted investigations, which, as we have argued in this book, may sometimes provide an appropriate way forward. For instance, it is not difficult to contemplate a test of pragmatic comprehension based on the ideas from relevance theory. The analysis of conversation also provides rich insight into children's pragmatic functioning, provided that the whole of the interaction is adequately considered and that some theoretical motivation is underpinning the analysis. Narratives have always been considered a valuable source of information on how children plan and execute plans, how they structure their thoughts, how they reflect on their environment and how they consider the needs of the reader/listener. Narratives have, of course, wider value as a window on children's linguistic skills in general. How language is used by children provides a unique window on their capabilities and impairments and, in the context of children's pragmatic impairments, how language is used is the defining feature of their impairment.

We hope to have demonstrated in this book that pragmatic functioning is intrinsically linked to cognitive functioning, both from the point of view of theory and research. In order to be able to produce pragmatically viable language and to comprehend beyond what is linguistically given, we need to think about the content and capabilities of the minds of others. We need to appraise what it is that others know and intend and what kind of information they are able to bring to the communication process at a particular point in time. In order to be able to process language in a communicative situation we need to be able to engage in inferential processing of the incoming information as we cannot simply rely on the linguistic expression itself for knowing the intended meaning. We also require world knowledge, and the ability to learn about the world in the first instance, in order to interpret meaning in context. We need to be able to relate utterances we hear (receive) to larger stretches of previous discourse, and not just to what is immediately preceding. We need to be capable of handling concepts that are divorced from the here and now. For the ability to use language in communication to develop, we need experience of communicative situations and human relationships. It may be that certain aspects of pragmatic functioning will be found to relate more closely to certain underlying abilities and hence a more fine-grained, and hopefully clinically helpful, view of children's pragmatic abilities will emerge.

References

Aarons M, Gittens T (1987) Is This Autism? Windsor: NFER-Nelson.

Adams C (1991) Analysis of language impaired children's conversation. In K Mogford-Bevan, J Sadler (eds) Child Language Disability II: Semantic and Pragmatic Difficullties. Clevedon: Multilingual Matters, pp.68–74.

Adams C, Bishop DVM (1989) Conversational characteristics of children with semantic-pragmatic disorder I: Exchange structure, turntaking, repairs and cohesion. British Journal of Disorders of Communication 24: 211–39.

American Psychiatric Association (1994) Diagnostic and Statistical Manual of Mental Disorders, 3rd revised edition (DSM-IV). Washington, DC: American Psychiatric Association.

Andersen-Wood L, Smith BR (1997) Working with Pragmatics. Bicester: Winslow Press.

Atkinson M (1979) Prerequisites for reference. In E Ochs, B Schieffelin (eds) Developmental Pragmatics. New York: Academic Press, pp.229–49.

Austin JL (1962) How to do Things with Words (2nd Edition). Oxford: Oxford University Press.

Baltaxe CAM, D'Angiola N (1996) Referencing skills in children with autism and specific language impairment. European Journal of Disorders of Communication 31: 245–58.

Bamberg M (1987) The Acquisition of Narratives. New York: Mouton de Gruyter.

Bamberg M, Damrad-Frye R (1991) On the ability to provide evaluative comments: Further explorations of children's narrative competencies. Journal of Child Language 18: 689–710.

Bates E (1976) Language and Context: The Acquisition of Pragmatics. New York: Academic Press.

Bates E (1979) The Emergence of Symbols: Cognition and Communication in Infancy. New York: Academic Press.

Bateson MC (1975) Mother-infant exchanges: The epigenesis of conversational interaction. In D Aaronson, RW Rieber (eds) Developmental Psycholinguistics and Communication Disorders. New York: Academy of Sciences, 18: 101–13.

de Beaugrande R, Dressler W (1981) Introduction to Text Linguistics. London: Longman.

Bennett-Kastor T (1983) Noun phrases and coherence in child narratives. Journal of Child Language 10: 135–49.

Bishop DVM (1979) Comprehension in developmental language disorders. Developmental Medicine and Child Neurology 21: 225–38.

Bishop DVM (1982) Comprehension of spoken, written and signed sentences in childhood language disorders. Journal of Child Psychology and Psychiatry 23: 1–20.

Bishop DVM (1989) Autism, Asperger's syndrome and semantic pragmatic disorder: Where are the boundaries? British Journal of Disorders of Communication 24: 107–21.

Bishop DVM (1991) The underlying nature of specific language impairment. Journal of Child Psychology and Psychiatry 35: 3–66.

Bishop DVM (1997) Uncommon Understanding: Development and Disorders of Language Comprehension in Children. Hove: Psychology Press.

Bishop DVM (1998) Development of the Children's Communication Checklist (CCC): A method for assessing qualitative aspects of communicative impairment in children. Journal of Child Psychology and Psychiatry 39(6): 879–91.

Bishop DVM, Adams C (1989) Conversational characteristics of children with semantic-pragmatic disorder II: What features lead to judgements of inappropriacy? British Journal of Disorders of Communication 24: 241–63.

Bishop DVM, Adams C (1991) What do referential communication tasks measure? A study of children with specific language impairment. Applied Psycholinguistics 12: 199–215.

Bishop DVM, Adams C (1992) Comprehension problems in children with specific language impairment: Literal and inferential meaning. Journal of Speech and Hearing Research 35: 119–29.

Bishop DVM, Edmundson A (1987) Language impaired 4 year olds: Distinguishing transient from persistent impairment. Journal of Speech and Hearing Disorders 52: 156–73.

Bishop DVM, Rosenbloom L (1987) Classification of childhood language disorders. In W Yule, M Rutter (eds) Language Development and Disorders: Clinics in Developmental Medicine. London: MacKeith Press, pp.16–41.

Bishop DVM, Chan J, Adams C, Hartley J, Weir F (in press) Conversational responsiveness in specific language impairment: Evidence of disproportionate pragmatic difficulties in a subset of children. Development and Psychopathology.

Bishop DVM, Hartley J, Weir F (1994) Why and when do some language impaired children seem talkative? A study of initiation in conversations of children with semantic-pragmatic disorder. Journal of Autism and Developmental Disorders 24(2): 177–97.

Blakemore D (1992) Understanding Utterances: An Introduction to Pragmatics. Oxford: Blackwell.

Botting N (1998) Semantic-pragmatic disorder as a distinct diagnostic entity: Making sense of the boundaries (a comment on Boucher). International Journal of Language and Communication Disorders 33(1): 71–108.

Botting N, Conti-Ramsden G (in press) Pragmatic language impairment without autism: The children in question. Autism.

Boucher J (1998a) SPD as a distinct diagnostic entity: Logical considerations and directions for future research. International Journal of Language and Communication Disorders 33(1): 71–81.

Boucher J (1998b) Some issues in the classification of developmental disorders. International Journal of Language and Communication Disorders 33(1): 95–108.

Bowler DM, Brook SL (1998) SPD and autistic spectrum disorder. International Journal of Language and Communication Disorders 33(1): 91–4.

Brook SL, Bowler DM (1992) Autism by another name? Semantic and pragmatic impairments in children. Journal of Autism and Developmental Disorders 22: 61–81.

Brown P, Levinson S (1987) Politeness: Some Universals in Language Usage. Cambridge: Cambridge University Press.

Bruner J (1990) Acts of Meaning. Cambridge, MA: Harvard University Press.

Chiat S (1986) Personal pronouns. In P Fletcher, M Garman (eds) Language Acquisition (2nd Edition). Cambridge: Cambridge University Press, pp.339–55.

Clark EV (1978) From gesture to word: On the natural history of deixis in language acquisition. In JS Bruner, A Garton (eds) Human Growth and Development. Oxford: Clarendon Press, pp 85–120.

Clezy G (1979) Modification of the Mother-Child Interchange in Language, Speech and Hearing. London: Edward Arnold.

Conti-Ramsden G, Crutchley A, Botting N (1997) The extent to which psychometric tests differentiate subgroups of children with SLI. Journal of Speech, Language and Hearing Research 40: 765–77.

Conti-Ramsden G, Dykins J (1991) Mother–child interactions with language impaired children and their siblings. British Journal of Disorders of Communication 26: 337–54.

Conti-Ramsden G, Gunn M (1986) The development of conversational disability: A case study. British Journal of Disorders of Communication 21: 339–51.

Cooper J, Moodley M, Reynell J (1978) Helping Language Development. London: Edward Arnold.

Coupe J, Goldbart J (1988) Communication Before Speech. London: Croom Helm.

Craig HK, Evans JL (1993) Pragmatics and SLI: Within-group variations in discourse behaviors. Journal of Speech and Hearing Research 36: 777–89.

Crais ER, Chapman RS (1987) Story recall and inferencing skills in language/learning-disabled and nondisabled children. Journal of Speech and Hearing Disorders 52: 50–5.

Crystal D, Davy D (1975) Advanced Conversational English. London: Longman.

Culloden M, Hyde-Wright S, Shipman A (1986) Non-syntactic features of 'semantic-pragmatic' disorders. In Advances in Working with Language Disordered Children. London: I CAN, pp.163–7.

Damico J (1985) Clinical discourse analysis. A functional approach to language assessment. In C Simon (ed.) Communication Skills and Classroom Success. San Diego, CA: College-Hill Press, pp.165–205.

Dewart H, Summers S (1995) Pragmatics Profile. Windsor: NFER-Nelson.

Dore J (1975) Holophrases, speech acts and language universals. Journal of Child Language 2: 21–40.

Dunn LM, Dunn LM, Whetton C, Burley J (1997) The British Picture Vocabulary Scale (2nd edition). Windsor: NFER-Nelson.

Edmondson W (1981) Spoken Discourse. London: Longman.

Eggins S, Slade D (1997) Analysing Casual Conversation. London: Cassell.

Ervin-Tripp S (1976) Is Sybil there? The structure of some American-English directives. Language in Society 5: 25–66.

Fey ME, Leonard LB (1983) Pragmatic skills of children with specific language impairment. In TM Gallagher, CA Prutting (eds) Pragmatic Assessment and Intervention Issues in Language. San Diego, CA: College-Hill Press, pp.65–82.

Fivush R, Gray JT, Fromhoff FA (1987) Two year olds talk about the past. Cognitive Development 2: 393–409.

Flavell JH (1985) Cognitive Development (2nd Edition). Englewood Cliffs, NJ: Prentice-Hall.

Fletcher M, Birt D (1983) Storylines. London: Longman.

Foster-Cohen SH, Konrad E (1996) 'If you'd like to burn your mouth feel free': A relevance theoretic account of conditionals used to children. In M Groefsema (ed.)

Proceedings of the University of Hertfordshire Relevance Theory Workshop. Chelmsford: Peter Thomas Associates.

Fryer A (1994) The Hanen early language parent programme. In J Law (ed.) Before School: A Handbook of Approaches to Intervention with Preschool Language Impaired Children. London: AFASIC, pp.1–18.

Gagnon L, Mottron L, Joanette Y (1997) Questioning the validity of the semantic-pragmatic syndrome diagnosis. Autism 1(1): 37–55.

Garvey C (1975) Requests and responses in children's speech. Journal of Child Language 2: 41–63.

German DJ (1986) Test of Word Finding. Allen, TX: DLM Teaching Resources.

Glucksberg S, Krauss RM (1967) What do people say after they have learned to talk? Studies of the development of referential communication. Merrill-Palmer Quarterly 13: 309–16.

Goody EN (1978) Towards a theory of questions. In E Goody (ed.) Questions and Politeness. Cambridge: Cambridge University Press, pp.17–43.

Grice P (1975) Logic and conversation. In P Cole, J Morgan (eds) Syntax and Semantics III: Speech Acts. New York: Academic Press, pp.41–58.

Grundy P (1995) Doing Pragmatics. London: Edward Arnold.

Halliday MAK (1975) Learning How to Mean. London: Edward Arnold.

Halliday MAK, Hasan R (1976) Cohesion in English. London: Longman.

Happé FGE (1993) Communicative competence and theory of mind in autism: A test of relevance theory. Cognition 48: 101–19.

Happé FGE (1994) Current psychological theories of autism: The theory of mind account and rival theories. Journal of Child Psychology and Psychiatry 35(2): 215–29.

Happé F (1995) Understanding minds and metaphors: Insights from the study of figurative language in autism. Metaphor and Symbolic Activities 10(4): 275–95.

Harris M (1992) Language Experience and Early Language Development. Hove: Lawrence Erlbaum Associates.

Hoey M (1991) Some properties of spoken discourses. In R Bowers, C Brumfit (eds) Applied Linguistics and English Language Teaching. London: Macmillan, pp.65–84.

Howell J, Dean E (1994) Treating Phonological Disorders in Children (2nd Edition). London: Whurr.

Hyde-Wright S, Cray B (1991) A teacher's and a speech therapist's approach to management. In K Mogford-Bevan, J Sadler (eds) Child Language Disability, Volume 2: Semantic and Pragmatic Difficulties. Clevedon: Multilingual Matters, pp.75–98.

Hymes D (1972) Models of the interaction of language and social life. In J Gumperz, D Hymes (eds) Directions in Sociolinguistics. New York: Rinehart and Winston, pp.35–71.

Johnston J, Smith LB (1989) Dimensional thinking in language impaired children. Journal of Speech and Hearing Research 32: 33–8.

Johnston JR, Smith LB, Box P (1997) Cognition and communication: Referential strategies used by preschoolers with specific language impairment. Journal of Speech, Language and Hearing Research 40: 964–74.

Jones S, Smedley M, Jennings M (1986) Case study: A child with a high level language disorder characterised by syntactic, semantic and pragmatic difficulties. In Advances in Working with Language Disordered Children. London: I CAN.

Jordan R (1989) An experimental comparison of the understanding and use of speaker-addressee personal pronouns in autistic children. British Journal of Disorders of Communication 24: 109–19.

Jordan R, Powell S (1995) Understanding and Teaching Children With Autism. Chichester: Wiley.

Kerbel D, Grunwell P (1998a) A study of idiom comprehension in children with semantic-pragmatic difficulties. Part 1: Task effects on the assessment of idiom comprehension in children. International Journal of Language and Communication Disorders 33(1): 1–22.

Kerbel D, Grunwell P (1998b) A study of idiom comprehension in children with semantic-pragmatic difficulties. Part 2: Between-groups results and discussion. International Journal of Language and Communication Disorders 33(1): 23–44.

King F (1989) Assessment of pragmatic skills. Child Language Teaching and Therapy 5: 191–201.

Kiss S (1996) Issues in developmental 'theory of mind' research from the point of view of relevance theory. In M Groefsema (ed.) Proceedings of the University of Hertfordshire Relevance Theory Workshop. Chelmsford, Peter Thomas Associates, pp.131–9.

Klecan-Aker JS (1993) A treatment programme for improving story-telling ability: A case study. Child Language Teaching and Therapy 9(2): 105–13.

Labov W, Fanshel D (1977) Therapeutic Discourse. London: Academic Press.

Leinonen E (1995) Children's pragmatic difficulties: Problems with context analysis? Finnish Journal of Logopedics and Phoniatrics 15(3–4): 87–96.

Leinonen E, Kerbel D (1999) Relevance theory and pragmatic impairment. International Journal of Language and Communication Disorders 34(4): 367–90.

Leinonen E, Letts CA (1997a) Referential communication tasks: Performance by normal and pragmatically impaired children. European Journal of Disorders of Communication 32: 53–65.

Leinonen E, Letts CA (1997b) Why pragmatic impairment? A case study in the comprehension of inferential meaning. European Journal of Disorders of Communication 32: 35–51.

Leinonen E, Letts C, Parke T (1994) Pragmatic impairment in children: A look at narratives. In R Aulanko, A-M Korpijaakko-Huuhka (eds) Proceedings of the Third Congress of the International Clinical Phonetics and Linguistics Association, University of Helsinki, pp.113–20.

Leinonen E, Smith BR (1994) Appropriacy judgements and pragmatic performance. European Journal of Disorders of Communication 29: 77–84.

Leinonen-Davies E (1988) Textual deviance in foreign learner compositions. In A Turney (ed.) Applied Text Linguistics. Exeter: Exeter University Press.

Letts CA (1985a) Aspects of Linguistic Interaction in Speech Therapy, Unpublished PhD thesis, Reading University.

Letts CA (1985b) Linguistic interaction in the clinic: How do therapists do therapy? Child Language Teaching and Therapy 1: 321–31.

Letts CA (1989) Exploring therapy and classroom interaction. In P Grunwell, A James (eds) The Functional Evaluation of Language Disorders. London: Croom Helm, pp.125–40.

Letts C (1991) The problem of reliability in the assessment of semantic-pragmatic disorder. In Proceedings of the Conference on Child Language Disorders, Norwegian Centre for Child Research. Report No. 24, Trondheim.

Letts CA, Rei J (1994) Using conversational data in the treatment of pragmatic disorder in children. Child Language Teaching and Therapy 10: 1–22.

Levinson S (1983) Pragmatics. Cambridge: Cambridge University Press.

Liles BZ (1985) Cohesion in the narratives of normal and language-disordered children. Journal of Speech and Hearing Research 28: 123–33.

Liles BZ (1987) Episode organisation and cohesive conjunctives in narratives of children with and without language disorders. Journal of Speech and Hearing Research 30: 185–96.

Liles BZ (1993) Narrative discourse in children with language disorders and children with normal language: A critical review of the literature. Journal of Speech and Hearing Research 36: 868–82.

Lloyd P (1990) Children's communication. In R Greve, M Hughes (eds) Understanding Children: Essays in Honour of Margaret Donaldson. Oxford: Blackwell, pp 51–70.

Lund NJ, Duchan JF (1993) Assessing Children's Language in Naturalistic Contexts (3rd Edition). Englewood Cliffs, NJ: Prentice Hall.

McCabe A, Peterson C (eds) (1991) Developing Narrative Structure. Hillsdale, NJ: Lawrence Erlbaum.

McLaughlin S (1998) Introduction to Language Development. San Diego, CA: Singular.

McTear M (1985a) Children's Conversation. Oxford: Blackwell.

McTear M (1985b) Pragmatic disorders: A case study of conversational disability. British Journal of Disorders of Communication 20: 129–33.

McTear M (1985c) Pragmatic disorders: A question of direction. British Journal of Disorders of Communication 10: 119–27.

McTear M, Conti-Ramsden G (1992) Pragmatic Disability in Children. London: Whurr.

Merritt DD, Liles BZ (1987) Story grammar ability in children with and without language disorder: Story generation, story retelling and story comprehension. Journal of Speech and Hearing Research 30: 539–51.

Merritt DD, Liles BZ (1989) Narrative analysis: Clinical applications of story generation and story retelling. Journal of Speech and Hearing Disorders 54: 438–47.

Mills A, Pulles A, Witten F (1992) Semantic and pragmatic problems in specifically language disordered children: One or two problems? Scandinavian Journal of Logopedics and Phoniatrics 17: 51–7.

Milosky LM (1992) Children listening: The role of world knowledge in language comprehension. In RS Chapman (ed.) Processes in Language Acquisition and Disorders. London: Mosby Year Book, pp.20-44.

Nelson K (1986) Event Knowledge. Hillsdale, NJ: Lawrence Erlbaum.

Nelson K (1989) Narratives from the Crib. Cambridge, MA: Harvard University Press.

Ninio A, Snow CE (1996) Pragmatic Development. Colorado: Westview Press.

Oakhill J (1984) Inferential and memory skills in children's comprehension of stories. British Journal of Educational Psychology 54: 31–9.

Oakhill J, Yuill N (1986) Pronoun resolution in skilled and less-skilled comprehenders: Effects of memory load and inferential complexity. Language and Speech 29: 25–37.

Oakhill J, Yuill N, Parkin A (1986) On the nature of the difference between skilled and less-skilled comprehenders. Journal of Research in Reading 9: 80–91.

Parnell MM, Amerman JD (1983) Answers to WH questions: Research and application. In TM Gallagher, CA Prutting (eds) Pragmatic Assessment and Intervention Issues in Language. San Diego, CA: College-Hill Press, pp.129–50.

Peterson C (1990) The who, when and where of early narratives. Journal of Child Language 17(2): 433–55.

Peterson C, Dodsworth P (1991) A longitudinal analysis of young children's cohesion and noun specification in narratives. Journal of Child Language 18: 397–415.

Piaget J (1926/1955) The Language and Thought of the Child. London: Routledge and Kegan Paul.

Prior M, Eisenmajer R, Leekam S, Wing L, Gould J, Ong B, Dowe D (1998) Are there subgroups within the autistic spectrum? A cluster analysis of a group of children with autistic spectrum disorders. Journal of Child Psychology and Psychiatry 39(6): 893–902.

Prutting C, Kirchner D (1983) Applied pragmatics. In T Gallagher, C Prutting (eds) Pragmatic Assessment and Intervention Issues in Language. San Diego, CA: College-Hill Press, pp.29–64.

Prutting C, Kirchner D (1987) A clinical appraisal of the pragmatic aspects of language. Journal of Speech and Hearing Disorders 52: 105–19.

Purcell S, Liles BZ (1992) Cohesion repairs in the narratives of normal-language and language disordered school-age children. Journal of Speech and Hearing Research 35: 354–62.

Rapin I, Allen DA (1983) Developmental Language Disorders: Nosologic Considerations. In U Kirk (ed.) Neuropsychology of Language, Reading and Spelling. London: Academic Press, pp.155–84.

Rapin I, Allen DA (1987) Developmental dysphasia and autism in preschool children: Characteristics and subtypes. In J Martin, P Fletcher, P Grunwell, D Hall (eds) Proceedings of the First Symposium of Specific Speech and Language Disorders in Children. London: AFASIC, pp.20–35.

Rapin I, Allen DA (1998) The semantic-pragmatic deficit disorder: Classification issues. International Journal of Language and Communication Disorders 33(1): 71–108.

Renfrew C (1969) The Bus Story. Oxford: Renfrew.

Renfrew C (1995) Word Finding Vocabulary Test (4th edition). Bicester: Winslow Press.

Rutter M, Andersen-Wood L, Beckett C, Bredenkamp D, Castle J, Groothues C, Kreppner J, Keaveney L, O'Connor TG, and the English and Romanian Adoptees (ERA) Study Team. (1999) Quasi-autistic patterns following severe early global deprivation. Journal of Child Psychology and Psychiatry 40(4): 537–49.

Sacks H, Schegloff EA, Jefferson G (1974) A simplest systematics for the organisation of turn-taking for conversation. Language 50: 696–735.

Schieffelin BB (1979) Getting it together: An ethnographic approach to the development of communicative competence. In E Ochs, BB Schieffelin (eds) Developmental Pragmatics. London: Academic Press, pp 73–108.

Searle J (1969) Speech Acts. Cambridge: Cambridge University Press.

Searle JR (1975) Indirect speech acts. In P Cole, JL Morgan (eds) Syntax and Semantics 3: Speech Acts. New York: Academic Press, pp.59–82.

Shields J, Varley R, Broks P, Simpson A (1996a) Social cognition in developmental language disorders and high-level autism. Developmental Medicine and Child Neurology 38: 487–95.

Shields J, Varley R, Broks P, Simpson A (1996b) Hemispheric function in developmental language disorders and high-level autism. Developmental Medicine and Child Neurology 38: 473–86.

Shulman BB (1985) Test of Pragmatic Skills. Arizona: Communication Skills Builders.

Sinclair JM, Coulthard RM (1975) Towards an Analysis of Discourse. London: Open University Press.

Smedley M (1989) Semantic-pragmatic language disorder: A description with some practical suggestions for teachers. Child Language Teaching and Therapy 5(2): 174–90.

Smith BR, Leinonen E (1992) Clinical Pragmatics: Unravelling the Complexities of Communicative Failure. London: Chapman and Hall.

Snow CE, Ferguson CA (1977) (eds) Talking to Children. Cambridge: Cambridge University Press.

Sperber D, Wilson D (1987) Precis of relevance. Behavioral and Brain Sciences 10(4): 736–54.

Sperber D, Wilson D (1995) Relevance: Communication and Cognition (2nd Edition). Oxford: Blackwell.

Stenstrom A-B (1994) An Introduction to Spoken Interaction. London: Longman.

Stubbs M (1986) Educational Linguistics. Oxford: Blackwell.

Tierney K, Cogher L (1994) Non-directive therapy. In J Law (ed.) Before School: A Handbook of Approaches to Intervention with Preschool Language Impaired Children. London: AFASIC, pp.62-76.

Tizard B, Hughes M (1984) Young Children Learning: Talking and Thinking at Home and School. London: Fontana.

Umstead RS, Leonard LB (1983) Children's resolution of pronominal reference in text. First Language 4: 73–84.

Vance M, Wells B (1994) The wrong end of the stick: Language impaired children's understanding of non-literal language. Child Language Teaching and Therapy 10: 23–46.

Ward S (in press) An investigation into the effectiveness of an early intervention method for delayed language development in young children. International Journal of Language and Communication Disorders 34: 243–64.

Weismer SE (1985) Constructive Comprehension Abilities Exhibited by Language-Disordered Children. Journal of Speech and Hearing Research 28: 175–84.

Wells G (1985) Language Development in the Pre-School Years. Cambridge: Cambridge University Press.

Wells G, Montgomery M (1981) Adult-child interaction at home and at school. In P French, M Maclure (eds) Adult-Child Conversation. London: Croom Helm, 210–43.

Willcox A, Mogford-Bevan K (1995) Assessing conversational disability. Clinical Linguistics and Phonetics 9: 235–54.

Wilson D, Sperber D (1981) On Grice's theory of conversation. In P Werth (ed.) Conversation and Discourse. London: Croom Helm, pp.155–78.

Wing L (1988) The continuum of autistic characteristics. In E Schopler, GB Mesibov (eds) Diagnosis and Assessment in Autism. New York: Plenum.

Index